4-13-11
$138.00

Color Atlas of Cone Beam Volumetric Imaging for Dental Applications

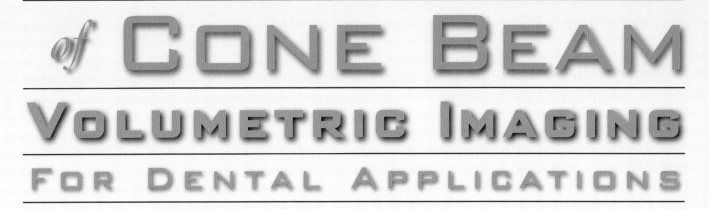

Color Atlas of Cone Beam Volumetric Imaging for Dental Applications

DALE A. MILES, DDS, MS

Oral and Maxillofacial Radiologist

Fountain Hills, Arizona

Quintessence Publishing Co, Inc

Chicago, Berlin, Tokyo, London, Paris, Milan, Barcelona, Istanbul, São Paulo, Mumbai, Moscow, Prague, and Warsaw

Library of Congress Cataloging-in-Publication Data

Miles, Dale A.
  Color atlas of cone beam volumetric imaging for dental applications / Dale
A. Miles.
      p. ; cm.
  Includes bibliographical references.
  ISBN 978-0-86715-481-8 (hardcover)
  1. Teeth--Tomography--Atlases. I. Title.
  [DNLM: 1. Cone-Beam Computed Tomography--methods--Atlases. 2.
Stomatognathic Diseases--radiography--Atlases. WN 17 M643c 2008]
  RK309.M56 2008
  617.60022'3--dc22

                                                    2008037989

© 2008 Quintessence Publishing Co, Inc

Quintessence Publishing Co Inc
4350 Chandler Drive
Hanover Park, IL 60133
www.quintpub.com

Editor: Bryn Goates
Design: Annette McQuade
Production: Sue Robinson

Printed in China

TABLE OF CONTENTS

PREFACE

Like any innovation in the dental profession, the availability of cone beam volumetric imaging (CBVI) has preceded understanding of its use. It happened with panoramic imaging as it did with digital radiographic imaging. The cone beam images in this atlas will educate dental professionals on how to use CBVI technology to better visualize the diseases and disorders that they encounter with their patients.

One aim of this atlas is to refresh the reader's memory of anatomy. As dentists, we never "worked" in the axial plane of section after our anatomy training; we have lived in a world of plain films or digital images, all in the format of 2-D grayscale panoramic, intraoral, or lateral cephalometric images. CBVI allows us to visualize patient anatomy and pathology like never before. With this technology we can not only view the patient's problems in three planes of section but colorize the image data sets in 3-D. CBVI helps to reveal bony changes caused by pathology. In addition, the level of anatomic detail in the 3-D image sets means that clinicians placing implants no longer have to experience anxiety about whether they are placed correctly. CBVI allows us to determine the precise location of the inferior alveolar nerve in relation to impacted mandibular third molars, which improves preoperative planning and reduces patient morbidity as well as our liability.

At last, we can see our patients' problems in a whole new manner—in 3-D and color. I hope this book helps you understand how CBVI can improve your clinical experiences and the management of your patients' treatment.

Acknowledgments

I am deeply appreciative to Mr Andrew Kim (CyberMed USA) and to Professor C. Young Kim (CyberMed International) for allowing me to beta test the initial software and to continue to use their product to image patient data sets to help readers visualize patient problems in a whole new light.

I would like to acknowledge Mr Bob Pienkowski and Mr Jim Fritz (Planmeca USA) for having the vision and patience to adopt this software and collaborate with CyberMed International to bring this technology to dentists and help us with our patients.

I would also like to thank the referring clinicians of Northwest Radiology in Seattle, Washington, for their confidence in my interpretive skills to serve their practice needs. This laboratory service, the clinicians they serve, and their wonderful patients have produced the data volumes that are featured in this text. Thanks to you all.

Thanks to Dr Ron Shelley for his help with my website. He represents the best of our profession, a dentist who cares about his patients and continually learns new techniques to help them with their dental problems.

Thanks also to Ms Tomoko Tsuchiya and Mr H. W. Haase, the publishers of Quintessence, for the opportunity to educate my colleagues about this incredible technology.

Finally, special thanks to my wife Kathryn for her support, love, confidence, sacrifice, and patience with me throughout my career and this project. I will make up the time, I promise.

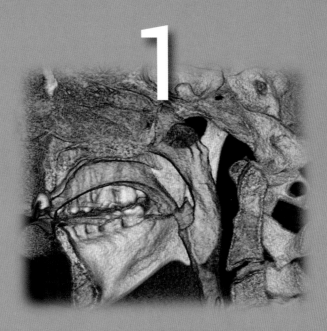

1

CONE BEAM VOLUMETRIC IMAGING IN CLINICAL PRACTICE

Nothing has captured the dental profession's imagination in the past few years like the introduction of cone beam volumetric imaging (CBVI), sometimes referred to as *cone beam computerized tomography* (CBCT) or *cone beam volumetric tomography* (CBVT). These machines' image acquisition process differs from that of traditional medical computerized tomography (CT) scanners in that the patient is not usually supine, the image gathered is in a voxel (volume element) format, the x-ray dose absorbed by the patient is substantially lower, appointment availability is much easier, and it is less expensive. In short, although the imaging modality produces significant data volumes like medical CT, it is vastly superior to traditional CT data for specific dental applications.

Box 1-1 Applications of CBVI

3-D virtual model construction

Airway studies related to sleep apnea

Bone structure (dehiscences, fenestrations, and/or periodontal defects in adults)

Impaction related to orthodontics

Implant site assessment including temporary anchorage devices

Inferior alveolar nerve location for third molar extraction

Odontogenic lesion visualization

Orthodontic assessment

Other computer-aided design/computer-assisted manufacture devices

Paranasal sinus evaluation

Space analysis (1:1)

Surgical guide fabrication

Temporomandibular joint visualization

Trauma evaluation

Dentists and dental specialists have seen and appreciated the incredibly precise and profound information produced by CBVI scans, and they are realizing that the data they receive will influence their treatment decisions like no other imaging modality used in the profession in the past 100 years. CBVI makes clinical decision making easier and more precise, patient treatment decisions more accurate, and visualization of the x-ray data more meaningful. Dentistry is moving away from "radiographic interpretation" and into "disease visualization," and it could not have come at a better time.

these are discussed in chapters 4 to 14. Additional applications will undoubtedly follow as clinicians learn about and begin to appreciate the incredibly beneficial data this imaging modality delivers for improved treatment planning and clinical decision making.

PRESENT CONSIDERATIONS FOR CBVI

THE NEAR FUTURE

The evolution of implant technology, the technical skills and training of dental professionals, and patients' desire for more permanent and predictable restorative solutions to missing teeth all ensure that implant dentistry will remain the largest growth market for dental professionals and commercial vendors for at least the next decade. I would predict that by 2013, the reconstructed data in 2-D/3-D grayscale and color formats from CBVI machines will become the standard of care for displaying patients' radiographic information in cases of preoperative implant site assessment, implant placement, and follow-up radiographic assessment. CT, plain film imaging, and digital imaging modalities will probably become obsolete, at least for implant dentistry applications.

The additional applications for CBVI encompass most of the procedures clinicians perform in their offices. Some applications for CBVI are listed in Box 1-1; examples of many of

To date, I have read, or interpreted, almost 3,000 CBVI cases for my dental colleagues. I practice my specialty of oral and maxillofacial radiology from my home in a dedicated radiology office environment via the Internet. I continue to interpret images and create reports for clinicians while I travel, speak, and consult. I operate in the same manner as my medical radiology colleagues and practice my specialty from virtually anywhere in the world because of global Internet access.

Just as there are many different models on the market, I receive data volumes to interpret through many different avenues. Gone are the days when we relied on 2-D grayscale single images attempting to represent 3-D structures, viewed on lightboxes under poor lighting conditions, to help us make our clinical treatment decisions. It is now possible to have 2-D or 3-D color "renderings" of each patient's anatomy and signs of clinical diseases/disorders.

Figure 1-1 shows the CBVI machine's broad capabilities and power. Whether you are considering purchasing a machine for image acquisition in your practice or are simply accessing this

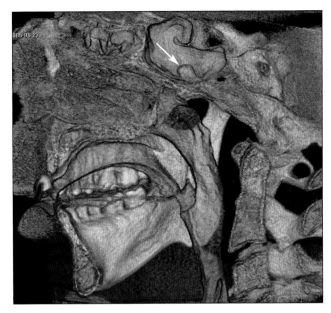

Fig 1-1 Large-volume 3-D color reconstruction of a patient's airway created with data from an i-CAT machine (Imaging Sciences International) and processed using Accurex software (CyberMed International). Note the cutaway sections of the mandible, the vertebral bodies, and the lesion in the sphenoid sinus, which is an osteoma. The color renderings aid in visualization of the soft tissue lining over the bony lesion (arrow).

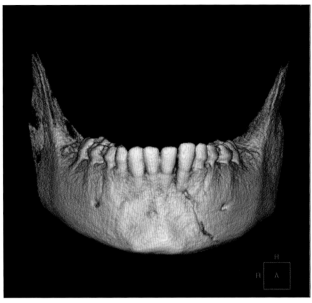

Fig 1-2 Small-volume 3-D color reconstruction of a 9-year-old patient with a fractured mandible, rendered with Accurex. The fracture is easily identified in the anteroposterior view, and the 3-D image can be rotated 360 degrees to see the fracture in any orientation.

3

technology by requesting a scan, you should consider the following important questions:

1. How much data (number of images) do you need?
2. How large an area do you wish to evaluate?
3. Do you need simple 2-D grayscale information for your decision?
4. Does the diagnostic task really require CVBI?
5. Does *every* patient require this type of imaging?
6. Are you comfortable diagnosing all of the data in the volume?
7. What is your risk of missing an important occult finding?

The data volume vs the single image

Before I address these questions, it is very important to understand the size difference between a data volume from a CBVI machine and traditional static 2-D grayscale images. Each periapical image on a computer is about 300 kB in size, and three of these static intraoral images would fill a 1-MB floppy disk. A digital panoramic image is about 5 to 7 MB, so approximately 100 images could fit on a CD-ROM. By contrast, each CBVI data volume acquired for a single patient can range from 100

to 250 MB. Only a few patient scans would fit on an 800-MB CD-ROM. Even the so-called small-volume machines provide much more anatomic information than we have been accustomed to viewing and assessing (Fig 1-2).

The impact of this data volume is huge, both literally and figuratively. Several large-capacity computers or servers are necessary to store the volumes. These data volumes should also be stored off-site via the Internet, which requires access to a high-speed Internet connection. As a clinician, remember that you are responsible for *all* of the information in the data volume, whether you order *or* acquire it, and whether for your own use or for a referral client. This is a fundamental paradigm shift for all clinicians that signals a move to the medical model of radiographic imaging; that is, we are shifting responsibility for the overall image findings to a qualified radiologist after more than 100 years of serving as our own radiology expert. Plain films and digital intraoral and panoramic images will still be used for some diagnostic procedures, but you will probably enlist the services of an oral and maxillofacial radiologist to look at your patients' data for occult pathology in anatomic regions that are less familiar to you. It is both prudent and professional to do so. Table 1-1 shows the reportable findings in 381 CBVI cases in a 1-year period (March 2005 to March 2006).

Table 1-1 Clinical findings of 381 CBVI reports*

Finding/ site of finding	Scanning service					Total
	CSP1	CSP2	Port	ADB	LVI	
Airway†	13	1	2	1	0	17
Bone‡	97	16	10	32	0	155
Dental	20	3	0	3	0	26
Nonodontogenic lesion§	4	0	0	0	0	4
Odontogenic lesion	20	1	1	5	0	27
Sinus	143	14	12	37	2	208
Soft tissue calcification	1	1	1	1	0	4
TMJ	39	10	5	13	0	67
Vertebral body‖	26	1	1	4	0	32
Other¶	78	19	3	27	2	129
Unremarkable	11	3	0	6	0	20
Total findings	**452**	**112**	**52**	**185**	**6**	**701**
No. of cases	**253**	**43**	**17**	**66**	**2**	**381**

*Several implants were reported impinging on anatomic spaces. One patient could not be scanned because of severe kyphosis. Gross caries lesions and periodontal bone loss were not tallied but were reported in the formal interpretive reports. Reprinted with permission from Miles DA.[1]
†Includes two cases of blocked ostium.
‡Includes apical periodontitis, residual cysts, furcations, recent extraction sites, impacted teeth, idiopathic osteosclerosis.
§Includes several antral lesions (extrinsic), a neurolemmoma, and a fractured zygoma.
‖Includes two surgical repairs: two cleft palate cases and one surgical nonunion case.
¶Includes congenitally missing teeth; calcified, elongated stylohyoid processes; calcified lymph nodes; retained roots; metallic fragments; hypoplasia/hyperplasia (facial, teeth); medial sigmoid depressions; dilacerated roots; tori; enostosis; submandibular salivary gland depressions; fibrous healing defects; two pharyngeal masses; and one possible case of Paget disease.
CSP1 = ClearScan Property (Phoenix, AZ); CSP2 = ClearScan Property (Peoria, AZ; lab service has since closed); Port = ClearScan Property (Portland, OR; lab service has since closed); ADB = Advanced Dental Board (Internet-based radiology reporting service); LVI = Las Vegas Institute (Las Vegas, NV); TMJ = temporomandibular joint.

Common CBVI concerns

How much data do you need?

This is very difficult to answer. Orthodontists or dentists who treat orthodontic problems in their patients require much more diagnostic information than other specialties to assess a case and predict the outcome. Currently, orthodontic assessment usually involves intraoral images; panoramic, cephalometric, and sometimes hand-wrist radiographs; and plaster casts. Casts are mentioned because, in the future, clinicians will create them from the radiographic data in the cone-beam scan. So the ability to acquire all of the image data needed in one single imaging procedure offers orthodontists a very distinct advantage over current methods. Of course, the clinician does not always need all of those images on an 8-year-old patient at the initial visit because it is unlikely that brackets will be placed on this patient until a few years later. Dentists should think about the information they need for each diagnostic task before they take or order a cone-beam scan. Known as *practicing by applying selection criteria*, this concept is only now becoming standard practice.[2]

How large an area do you wish to evaluate?

Some CBVI machines acquire larger data volumes than others. Data acquisitions range from volumes of 4 × 4 cm² to 22 × 22 cm². Figure 1-3 demonstrates the differences in size and region of the head corresponding to these volumes. Not all clinicians need to see the entire skull or would wish to be re-

Fig 1-3 Comparison between the results from a small-volume machine and those from a large-volume machine. *(top)* Axial slice of the middle of the condylar head. *(bottom)* Larger area at approximately the same level. Both volumes contain anatomic structures and cells, such as the middle ear, mastoid cells, airway, and vertebral bodies, all of which would require evaluation to determine whether pathology was present.

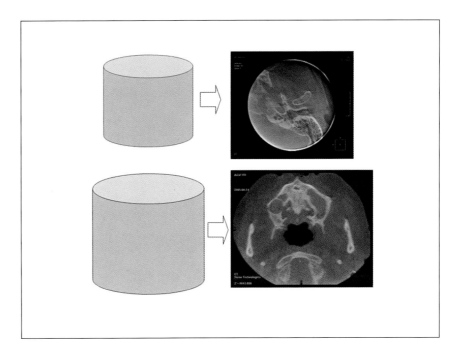

Fig 1-4 Digital panoramic radiograph of a developing mixed dentition. Except for the slightly ectopic resorption of the primary canine roots, the dentition is developing normally. This child would not need a cone beam scan to make this determination. The x-ray dose from the CBVI scan would *not* be justified simply to obtain this panoramic image.

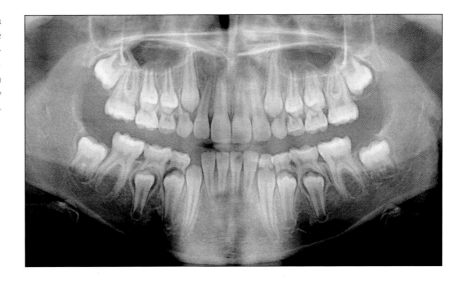

5

sponsible for the occult pathology that might be encountered in the data volume (slice). Radiologists and others wishing to assess a patient's data volume must scroll through and be able to detect pathologic findings in as many as 512 slices (images) in three orthogonal planes (axial, sagittal, and coronal). Most clinicians are not comfortable with this task or do not have the time to look at such a large amount of information.

Do you need simple 2-D grayscale information for your decision?
It may not be necessary to have 3-D color information for decision making at all. The reconstruction of a panoramic image from a 250-MB data volume requires anywhere from 4 to 70 times the amount of x-rays needed for a traditional panoramic

radiograph or digital image.[2] Therefore, a 2-D digital panoramic radiograph from a full-featured panoramic machine can often suffice for the preliminary visualization of the patient's dentition, bone, condyles, and related anatomy (Fig 1-4).

Does the diagnostic task really require CBVI?
The clinician must determine if CBVI is even necessary for a particular diagnostic task. Applications and clinical indications to help with this determination are discussed in later chapters. Detection of caries lesions does not require a cone-beam scan. Periodontal bone loss can be evaluated by well-positioned bitewing and periapical radiographs. Some underestimation of the alveolar architecture may occur in plain film or digital intraoral radiography, but this task still does not require CBVI's

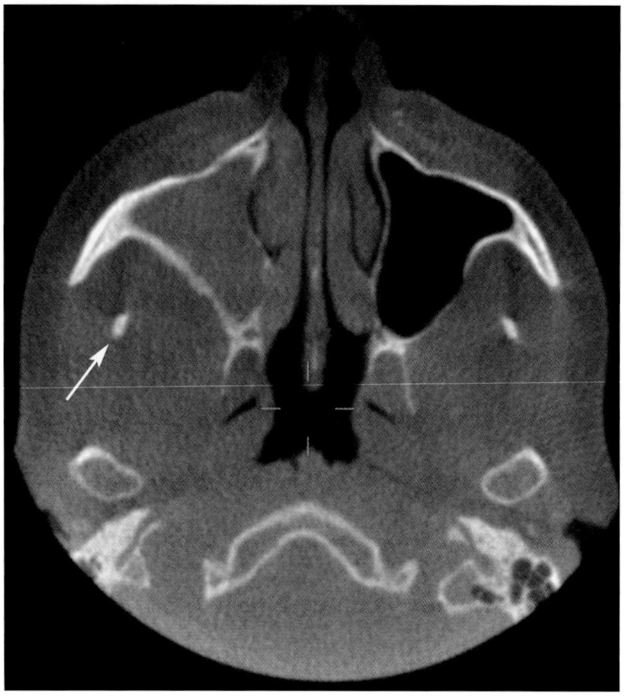

Fig 1-5 Try to identify the structure designated by the *white arrow*, but do not be surprised if you do not recognize it; most dentists have never seen this structure in this plane of section. Note the total opacification of the right maxillary sinus. As is conventionally done in medical CT and with panoramic radiographs, we are viewing the patient from the foot end, so the patient's right side is the left side of the image. The indicated structure is the coronoid process.

thin slice data to see bone problems. If a patient exhibits a systemic disease or a set of risk factors that could accelerate the bone loss associated with periodontal disease, a cone-beam scan may be indicated to detect the disease earlier or monitor the treatment success. However, noninvasive, diagnostic immunoassay tests performed on saliva could detect disease processes even earlier without exposing the patient to any x-rays. The clinician should carefully consider the precise indications for this imaging modality and fully expect the images produced to result in a positive finding that could affect a treatment outcome. Although x-ray doses are lower for any CBVI machine than traditional medical CT, not every patient will require a cone beam scan.[2]

Does every patient require this type of imaging?

The short answer is an emphatic *no*. Again, the clinician must consider the application and prescribe this imaging test only for those patients who would actually benefit from a precise measurement for an implant site or a better outcome prediction based on the data volume acquired. There are enough reasons to use CBVI.[1,4] Income generation is *not* one of them, nor is the production of "prettier images."

Are you comfortable diagnosing all of the data in the volume?

Most clinicians are not comfortable viewing radiographic data in an axial plane. Anatomic structures and pathology in a thin slice format, which only displays a plane of information 1 mm thick (or less), are rare. Consider the image in Fig 1-5 and ask yourself if you can identify the structure indicated by the white arrow.

What is your risk of missing an important occult finding?

There is a lot of interest and some confusion regarding who is responsible for the image data in the CBVI volume. Is it the owner of the machine? Is it the referring doctor? Is it the specialist whose office has the machine and provides the radiographic data volume? The short answer is *yes*. Everyone in these various scenarios is liable. The dentist, the dental specialist who only provides images, and the radiographic imaging laboratory providing services for the referring clinician would all be named in a lawsuit if a significant finding were missed that resulted in harm to the patient. The only solution is to look at all of the images in all planes of section and record any abnormality. Then refer the patient, with the images, for a consultation with the appropriate clinician. If you do not feel capable of detecting and interpreting the data, or if you do not have the time, you should probably consider using a "reading service," medical or dental, to review the image data set and report the findings. There are always many reportable findings in CBVI scans.[1]

REFERENCES

1. Miles DA. Clinical experience with cone beam volumetric imaging: Report of findings in 381 cases. US Dent 2006;Sep:39–42.

2. US Department of Health and Human Services, Public Health Service, Food and Drug Administration; and American Dental Association, Council on Dental Benefit Programs, Council on Dental Practice, Council on Scientific Affairs. The selection of patients for dental radiographic examinations. Revised 2004. Available at: www.ada.org/prof/resources/topics/topics_radiography_examinations.pdf. Accessed 30 June 2008.

3. Ludlow JB, Davies-Ludlow LE, Brooks SL. Dosimetry of two extraoral direct digital imaging devices: NewTom cone beam CT and Orthophos Plus DS panoramic unit. Dentomaxillofac Radiol 2003;32:229–234.

4. Danforth RA, Miles DA. Cone beam volume imaging (CBVI): 3D applications for dentistry. Ir Dent 2007;10(9):14–18.

2

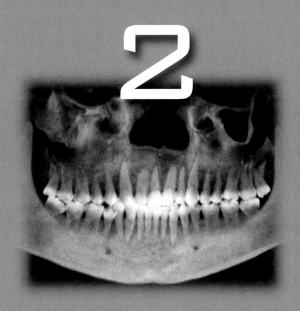

BASIC PRINCIPLES

The method of obtaining the patient's data volume in *cone beam volumetric imaging* (CBVI) differs significantly from that of conventional medical *computerized tomography* (CT). In medical CT scanning (previously termed *CAT [computed axial tomography]*), the patient's region of interest (ROI), such as the head or abdomen or other body part, is selected. As the x-ray source rotates around the ROI 60 times per minute, multiple sensors, consisting of either a gas or scintillator material, most commonly cesium iodide (CsI), detect the x-ray beam. The patient must be moved into the scanner a known distance in the z-plane. It is this distance—perhaps a centimeter, a half centimeter, or, in cases where higher resolution is required, as little as one millimeter—that determines the *slice thickness*. This type of image acquisition is very precise. The data acquired are voluminous and, in turn, the patient's absorbed x-ray dose is also very large. A typical CT scan for a maxillary implant site assessment may have a radiation dose as high as 2,100 µSv, equivalent to the dose from about 375 panoramic radiographic film or digital images.[1]

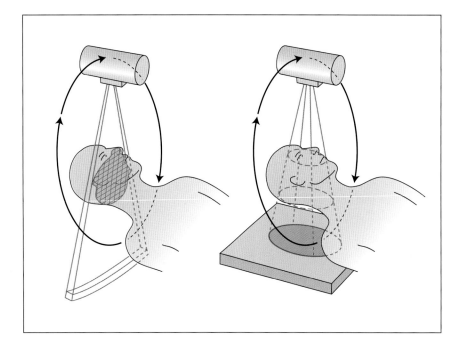

Fig 2-1 *(left)* A traditional medical CT detector array with x-ray source rotates 360 degrees around the patient about 60 times per minute. The thickness of each image slice is determined by the distance (usually 1.0 mm to 10.0 cm) the patient is moved through the gantry. This exposes the patient to a large dose of x-rays. *(right)* A cone beam device, using the cone-shaped beam, rotates around the patient. The exposure factors are similar to those used for exposing traditional dental x-rays, so the x-ray dose to the patient is substantially reduced compared to that of traditional medical CT.

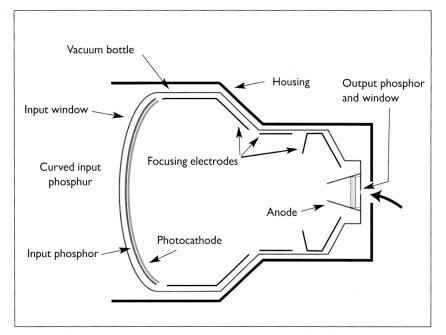

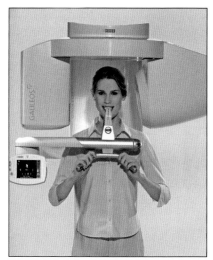

Fig 2-2a In the image intensification (II) system, a curved input phosphor, usually CSI, introduces geometric distortion, which must be compensated for by software. The phosphor coating will degrade over time, so the II will have to be replaced eventually—sometimes in as few as 3 or 4 years. This older imaging system is being replaced by flat-panel displays, which offer the many advantages of a direct digital capture.

Fig 2-2b This II system is stylish but large because of the II configuration. The x-ray source is on the left of the patient. The detector system is on the right side. (Courtesy of Sirona USA.)

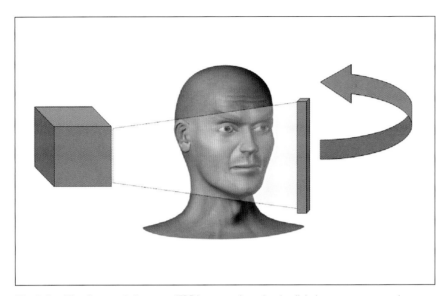

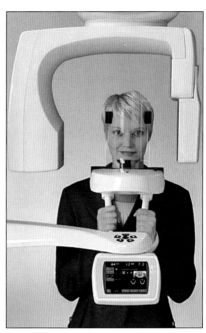

Fig 2-3a The flat-panel detector (FPD) system is a simple digital capture system that uses only an x-ray source and a digital detector to capture the image volume. The devices made with this type of system are much less bulky and therefore more ergonomic.

Fig 2-3b This FPD system is the ProMax 3D (Planmeca USA). (Courtesy of Planmeca USA.)

Image Acquisition

Unlike conventional CT, CBVI uses a narrow cone-shaped beam to rotate 194 to 360 degrees around the patient (Fig 2-1). The sensor is either an image intensifier (II) that is coupled to either a charge-coupled device (CCD) (Figs 2-2a and 2-2b) or complementary metal oxide semiconductor (CMOS), or a thin film transistor (TFT) flat-panel type of image receptor (Figs 2-3a and 2-3b). The II is older technology that was developed to improve the viewing of fluoroscopic images in the operating room during surgery. In the past, the bright lights of the operating room made it a poor environment for surgeons to view radiographic film, necessitating a device to "intensify" the resulting images. The major disadvantage of the II is distortion at the periphery of these systems. The image pattern appears as a sphere or "ball" and thus the edge regions are not ideal.

Flat-panel detectors (FPDs) are the newest image receptors for solid-state large area arrays.[2] These panels are expensive but offer some advantages over the older II systems including less distortion, wider scale of contrast, and elimination of veiling glare.

Compared to medical CT, CBVI doses are only about 40 to 500 µSv.[1] The method of acquiring images is very different and the exposure factors (kV and mA) are much lower. CBVI de-

vices use either a single FPD or an II (scintillator or phosphor screen) coupled to a series of CCDs. Table 2-1 illustrates the various machine parameters for the current CBVI devices. More information about CCDs is available at the LearnDigital website.[3]

Pixel vs Voxel Information

A pixel is a picture element. It is a square that measures between 20 and 60 µm in size. The size of the receptor area is the same whether it resides in an intraoral device, the TFT screen, or the II and solid-state combination device. CCDs and CMOSs for intraoral sensors are megapixel arrays, meaning that each is one million pixels or more. The larger flat panels, of course, use many millions of pixels.

A voxel is a volume element. This means that the pixel has a third side; it is really a cubed array. In CBVI, this cube is made up of isotropic pixels with equal sides. In conventional medical CT, the pixel is nonisotropic, meaning that two sides are equal but the third (z-plane) is a selectable width, anywhere from 0.5 mm to 1.0 cm or more. Figure 2-4 illustrates this difference.

Table 2-1 Characteristics of current CBVI machines

Scanner name	Manufacturer	Detector type	Maximum detector size (cm)	Voxel size (mm³)	Scan time (s)
3D Accuitomo	J. Morita USA	FPD	6.0 × 6.0	0.125	18
CB MercuRay	Hitachi Medical Systems America	II/CCD	10.2 × 19.0	0.200–0.380	10
Galileos	Sirona USA	II/CCD	15.0 × 15.0	0.150–0.300	14
i-CAT	Imaging Sciences International	FPD	20.0 × 25.0	0.120–0.400	5–25
Iluma	IMTEC	FPD	19.0 × 24.0	0.090–0.400	10–40
NewTom VG	AFP Imaging	FPD	15.0 × 16.0	0.160–0.320	20
PreXion 3D	TeraRecon	FPD	8.0 × 8.0	0.200	19–37
ProMax 3D	Planmeca USA	FPD	8.0 × 8.0	0.160	16–18
Scanora 3D	PaloDEx	FPD	7.5 × 14.5	0.150–0.350	20

*The Galileos, i-CAT, and ProMax 3D use a pulsed exposure, which turns the radiation source off and on at intervals. This lowers the overall absorbed radiation dose substantially.

†Only machines with comparable dose data that have been cited in recently published sources have been included.[4,5] ProMax 3D data are from personal communication (Kortesniemi M, 2008).

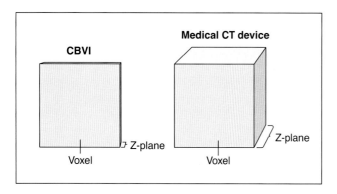

Fig 2-4 Traditional medical CT scanners use pixels. The slice thickness is determined by gantry movement. The thickness, or z-plane, is determined by the machine operator. CBVI devices gather the volume information directly using voxels or cubes with known dimensions (typically 0.15 mm to 0.60 mm). All CBVI slice thicknesses in the resulting data volume are much thinner than slices created by medical CT devices.

RADIATION DOSE

Although the radiation dose from CBVI machines is significant, it is much less than that of traditional medical CT scans. Recent data from Ludlow et al[1] estimates that the absorbed x-ray dose from a CBVI examination for a procedure such as an implant site assessment is between 1% and 25% the dose absorbed from a medical CT scan. This means that many dental-specific evaluations can be performed much more safely with CBVI than with medical CT. Thus, for any of the applications cited in Box 1-1 being considered for your patients, you cannot justify a medical CT procedure since its radiation dose would greatly exceed that of a CBVI evaluation (see Table 2-1). As more machines become available, more dose data are sure to follow. CBVI will become the imaging modality of choice for most dental tasks requiring 2-D/3-D information for clinical decision making.

Exposure time* (s)	Effective dose† (μSv)	Reconstruction time (min)	kV	mA	Focal spot	Weight (lb)
18.0	–	5.0	60–80	1.0–10.0	0.5	882
10.0	–	6.0	60–120	10.0–15.0	–	2000
14.0	39	4.5	85	5.0–7.0	–	352
3.0–8.0	61	<1.0	120	1.0–3.0	0.5	–
10.0–40.0	–	4.0 at 0.4 voxel	120	3.8	0.3	770
5.4	36.9	3.0	110	15.0	0.3	550
19.0	–	–	90	4.0	0.6	–
6.0	45	<3.0	84	12.0	0.5	248
5.0	–	3.0	85	8.0	0.4	690

13

LEGAL CONCERNS

A few of my colleagues believe, or have been advised by CBVI machine manufacturers, that they can simply have their patient sign a consent form stating that the dentist, because he/she is not sufficiently trained to interpret the data beyond the "dental bases," is not to be held liable if a significant finding is missed. Actually, both the owner of the CBVI machine and the referring clinician have a co-responsibility to make sure the entire data volume is reviewed for occult pathology. If they are not comfortable interpreting the volume, it is up to them to make sure a qualified individual reads the volume and reports the findings to them. *There is no ignoring this responsibility.*

Consider a lawyer questioning a machine owner on a witness stand. The following is a hypothetic conversation, but I assure you it is a reasonable line of inquiry.

Lawyer: Doctor X, was Miss Y present in your office on June 30, 2006, for an appointment to have a cone beam CT examination performed?

Doctor X: Yes.

Lawyer: And, Doctor X, was that cone beam CT examination actually performed?

Doctor X: Yes.

Lawyer: And, Doctor X, did you charge a fee for that cone beam CT examination?

Doctor X: Yes.

Lawyer: Doctor X, what was the fee you charged Miss Y for said cone beam CT examination?

Doctor X: Four hundred twenty-five dollars.

Lawyer: Doctor X, did you collect that fee from Miss Y?

Doctor X: Yes.

Lawyer: Well, Doctor X, wouldn't you call that "practicing dentistry"?

Doctor X: Yes, but . . .

Lawyer: Doctor X, just answer the question yes or no.

Doctor X: Yes.

As this fictional scenario demonstrates, when a clinician performs a procedure, charges a fee, and collects that fee, it is considered practicing dentistry. There is no other recourse than to ensure the images in the data volume are reviewed—all 512 images in each of the three orthogonal planes: axial, sagittal, and coronal. If you do not feel qualified to do this, it is essential to have that volume read by an oral and maxillofacial radiologist or a medical radiologist colleague.

REFERENCES

1. Ludlow JB, Davies-Ludlow LE, Brooks SL. Dosimetry of two extraoral direct digital imaging devices: NewTom cone beam CT and Orthophos Plus DS panoramic unit. Dentomaxillofac Radiol 2003 32:229–234.

2. Floyd P, Palmer P, Palmer R. Radiographic techniques. Br Dent J 1999: 187:359–365.

3. Miles DA. LearnDigital website. Available at: http://www.learndigital.net. Accessed 14 July 2008.

4. Hirsch E, Silva M. Radiation doses from different cone-beam-ct devices. Presented at the 11th Congress of the European Academy of Dento-Maxillo-Facial Radiology, Budapest, 27 Jun 2008.

5. Brooks SL. Answer to question #6120 submitted to "Ask the Experts." Health Physics Society website. Available at: http://hps.org/publicinformation/ate/q6120.html. Accessed 14 July 2008.

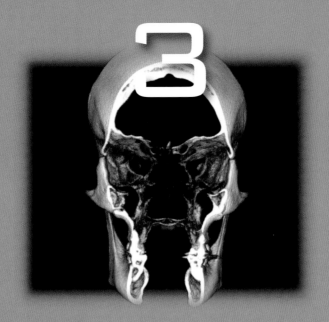

ANATOMIC STRUCTURES

To discern a potential problem in the cone beam volumetric imaging (CBVI) data volume, the clinician or radiologist must examine multiple slices in three planes of section: axial, sagittal, and coronal. While clinicians are quite familiar with many structures in the sagittal plane (since it is similar to periapical, bitewing, panoramic, and cephalometric orientations), they are not as familiar with these same structures as viewed in the coronal or especially the axial plane. To illustrate this point, I would ask you to look back at Fig 1-5 and recall the difficulty of interpreting thin slice data in a plane of section most of us have not seen since dental school.

This chapter presents many anatomic structures in the three planes of section as grayscale images, supported in most cases by thicker 3-D slices, slabs, or volume images to help readers orient themselves and recreate the structures in the mind's eye. No attempt was made to illustrate all structures; the chapter instead focuses on those that are commonly seen by dentists and dental specialists to help them relearn anatomic detail that may be long forgotten. Because many of the structures involve several bones, they are repeated in various views and planes of section.

15

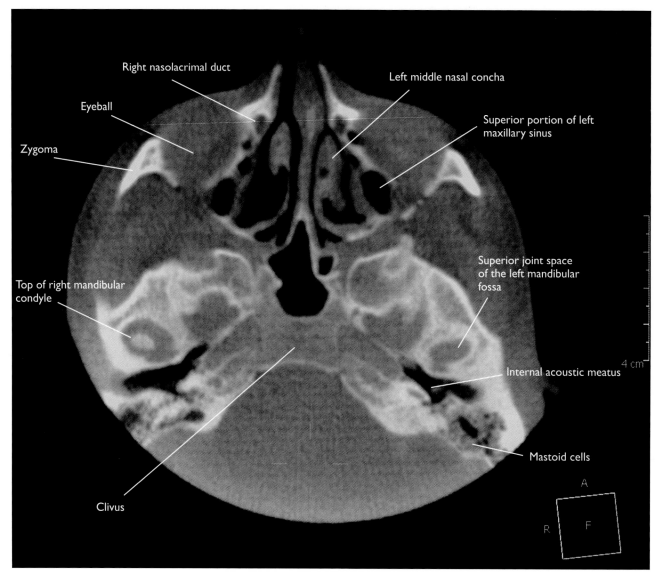

Right nasolacrimal duct

Left middle nasal concha

Eyeball

Superior portion of left
maxillary sinus

Zygoma

Superior joint space
of the left mandibular
fossa

Top of right mandibular
condyle

4 cm

Internal acoustic meatus

Mastoid cells

Clivus

Fig 3-1 A 0.15-mm slice at the level of the mandibular fossa (top of condyle).

MAXILLARY, NASAL, LACRIMAL, PALATINE, AND SPHENOID STRUCTURES

Maxillary structures should be very familiar to all of us, especially in the lateral or sagittal view. Although these bones can be described separately, we will see them in this chapter as they appear clinically—joined together to make walls, spaces, and structures that we must recognize to understand the 3-D changes one might encounter during an examination of a cone beam data volume. When possible, these structures will be identified as they relate to one another.

Structures identified in Figs 3-1 through 3-29 include the antra, incisive foramen and canal, nasal fossa, nasal conchae, nasolacrimal canal, pterygoid plates/processes, pterygoid hamu-

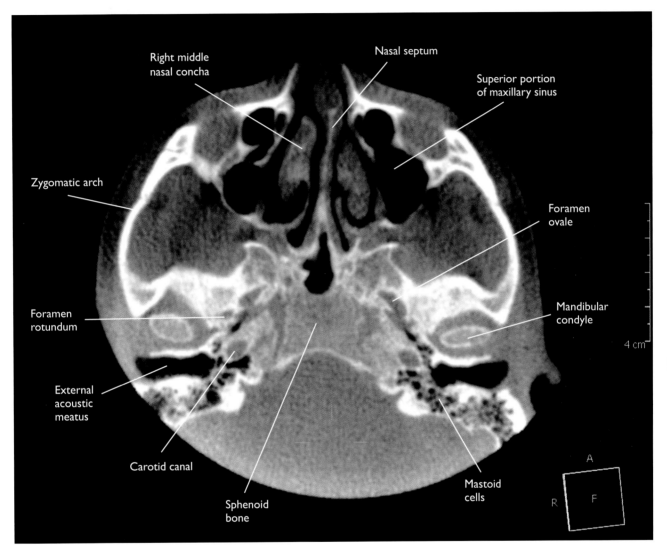

Fig 3-2 A 1-mm slice at the level of the mandibular fossa (middle of condyle).

lus, and styloid and mastoid processes. In each section, the structures are identified in the axial plane first (both thin and thick sections), followed by similar views in the sagittal and coronal planes. All three planes appear in Fig 3-29 to show the clinician and student how a specific structure or anomaly is oriented between the three planes. In most instances, the images start with a section through a recognizable part of the anatomy such as the temporomandibular joint (TMJ) condyles.

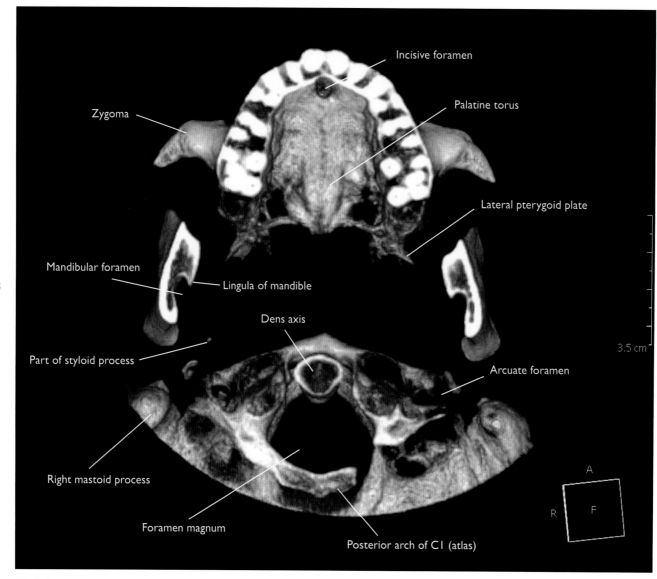

Incisive foramen

Palatine torus

Zygoma

Lateral pterygoid plate

Mandibular foramen

Lingula of mandible

Dens axis

Part of styloid process

Arcuate foramen

Right mastoid process

Foramen magnum

Posterior arch of C1 (atlas)

3.5 cm

A

R F

Fig 3-3 A 21.5-mm slice from the palatal to midportion of condyle.

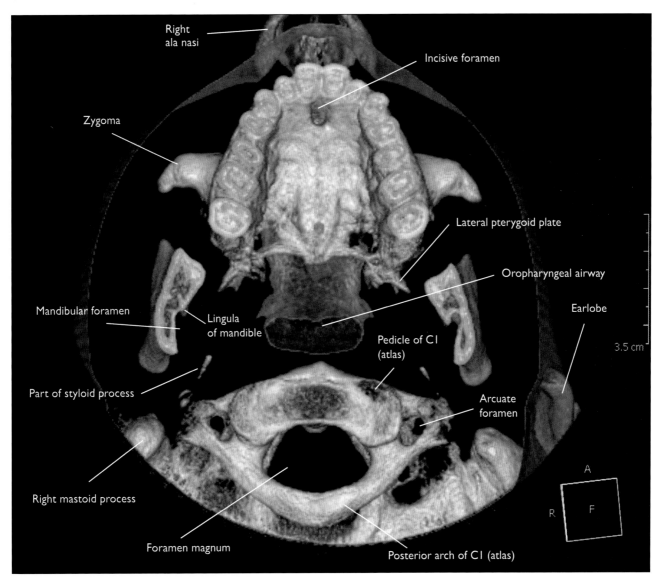

Right
ala nasi

Incisive foramen

Zygoma

Lateral pterygoid plate

Oropharyngeal airway

Mandibular foramen

Lingula
of mandible

Earlobe

3.5 cm

Pedicle of CI
(atlas)

Part of styloid process

Arcuate
foramen

Right mastoid process

A

R   F

Foramen magnum

Posterior arch of CI (atlas)

Fig 3-4 Same slice as shown in Fig 3-3, processed to show airway structures.

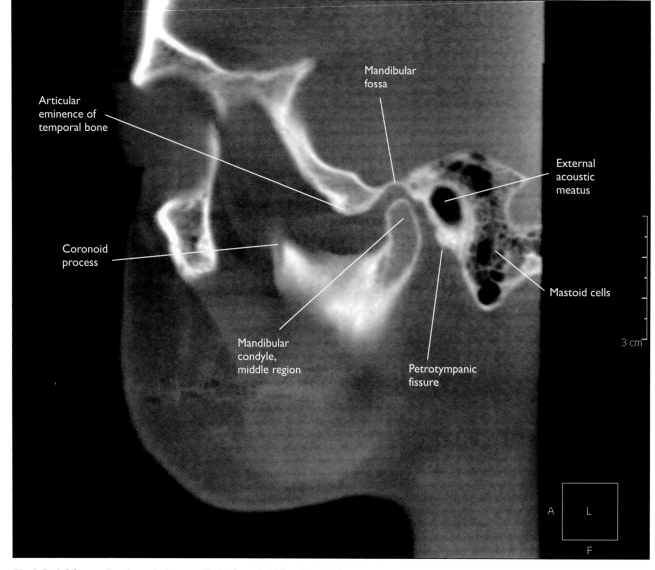

Articular
eminence of
temporal bone

Mandibular
fossa

Coronoid
process

External
acoustic
meatus

Mandibular
condyle,
middle region

Petrotympanic
fissure

Mastoid cells

3 cm

A L F

Fig 3-5 A 2.2-mm slice through the mandibular fossa (middle of condyle).

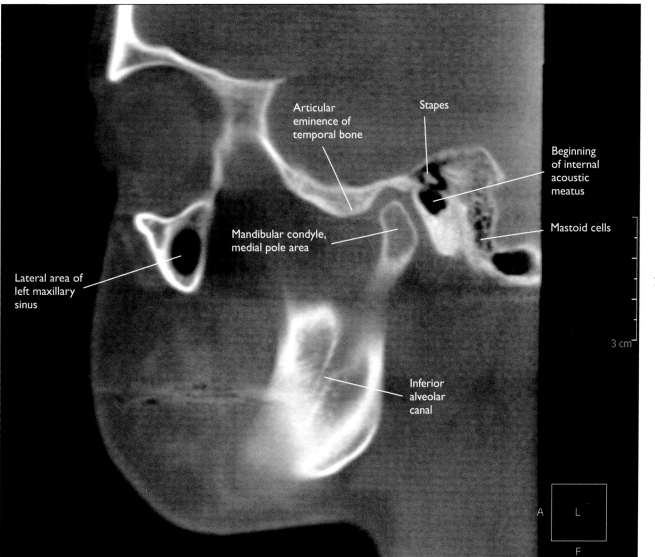

Fig 3-6 A 0.15-mm slice through the mandibular fossa (medial pole of condyle).

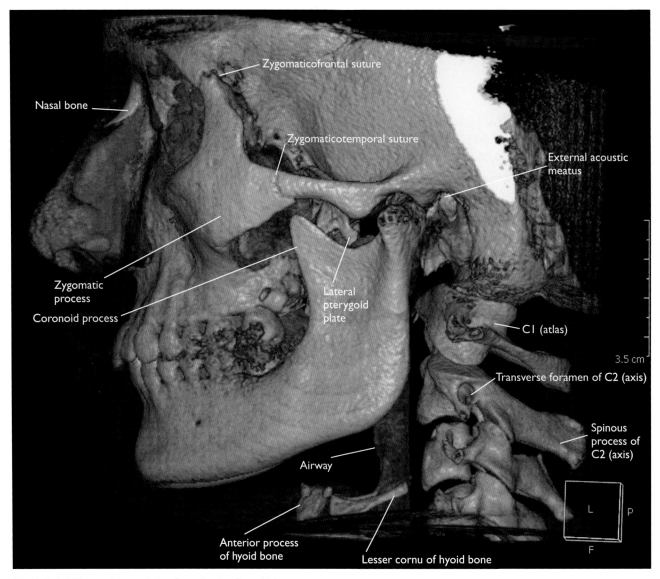

Fig 3-7 A 100-mm slab rendering (lateral pole of condyle).

Zygomaticofrontal suture

Nasal bone

Zygomaticotemporal suture

External acoustic meatus

Zygomatic process

Coronoid process

Lateral pterygoid plate

C1 (atlas)

3.5 cm

Transverse foramen of C2 (axis)

Spinous process of C2 (axis)

Airway

L   P

F

Anterior process of hyoid bone

Lesser cornu of hyoid bone

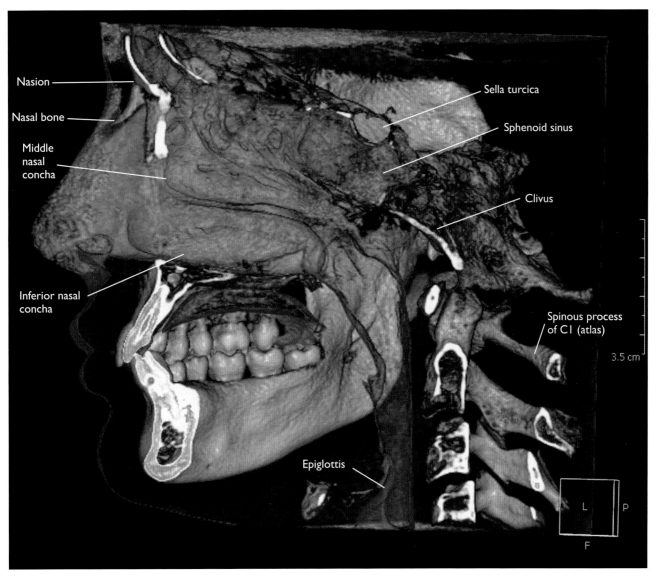

Nasion

Nasal bone

Middle
nasal
concha

Inferior nasal
concha

Sella turcica

Sphenoid sinus

Clivus

Spinous process
of C1 (atlas)

3.5 cm

Epiglottis

23

Fig 3-8 A 60-mm slab rendering (middle of condyle).

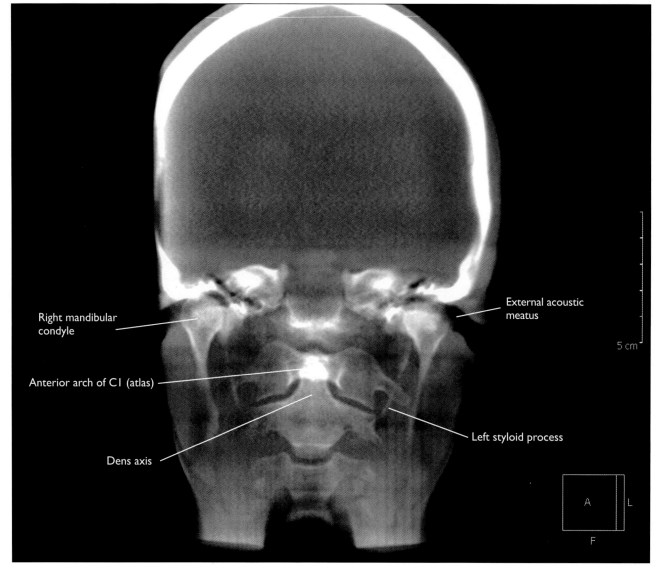

Right mandibular condyle

External acoustic meatus

Anterior arch of CI (atlas)

5 cm

Left styloid process

Dens axis

A

L

F

Fig 3-9 This 13.2-mm slice serves as a pseudoradiograph of the posterior region of the condyles.

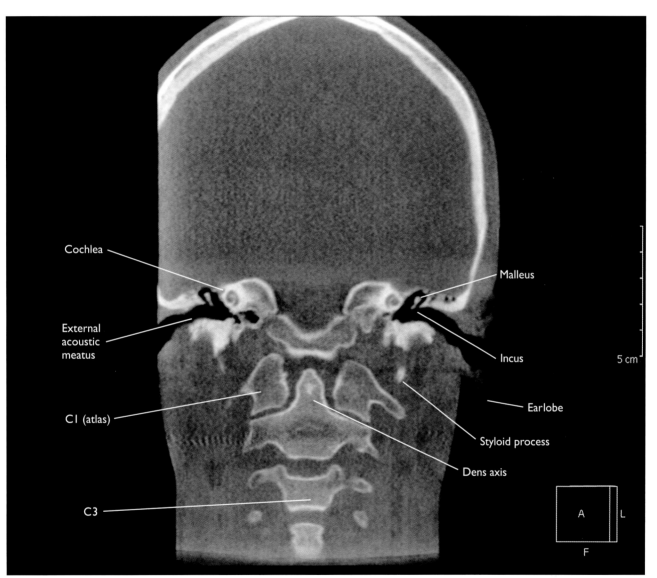

Fig 3-10 A 0.15-mm slice through the middle ear region.

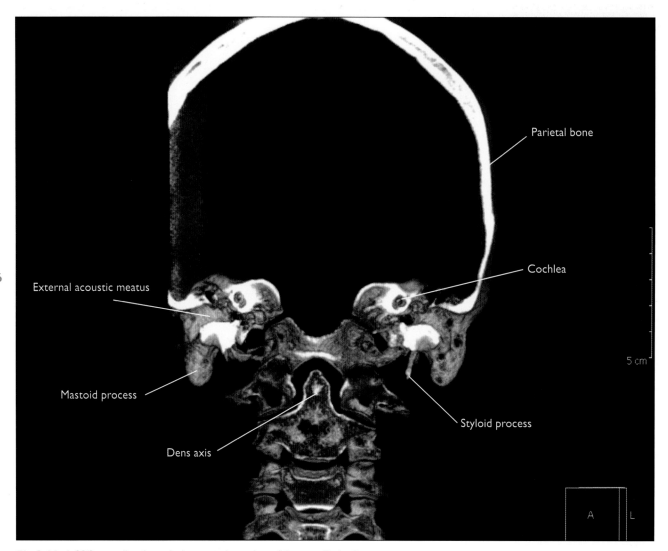

Parietal bone

Cochlea

External acoustic meatus

Mastoid process

Styloid process

Dens axis

5 cm

A   L

Fig 3-11 A 33.2-mm slice through the posterior region of the mandibular fossa.

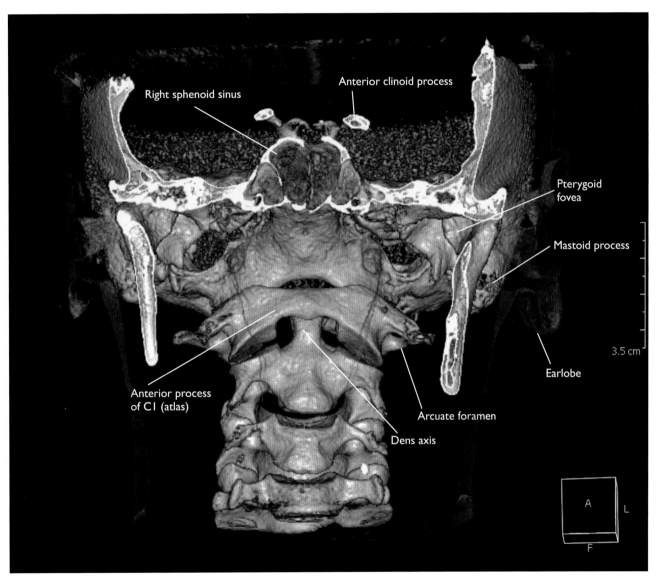

Fig 3-12 A 100-mm slice through the mandibular fossa.

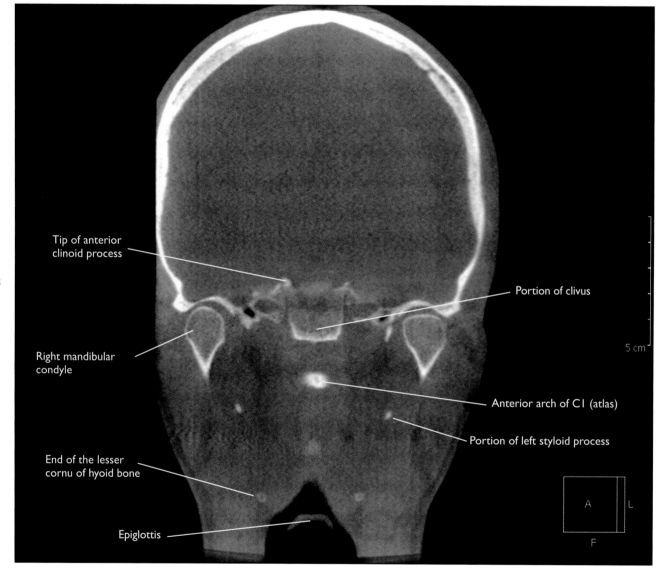

Tip of anterior clinoid process

Portion of clivus

5 cm

Right mandibular condyle

Anterior arch of C1 (atlas)

Portion of left styloid process

End of the lesser cornu of hyoid bone

A   L

F

Epiglottis

Fig 3-13 A 0.15-mm slice through the mandibular fossa (middle of the condyles).

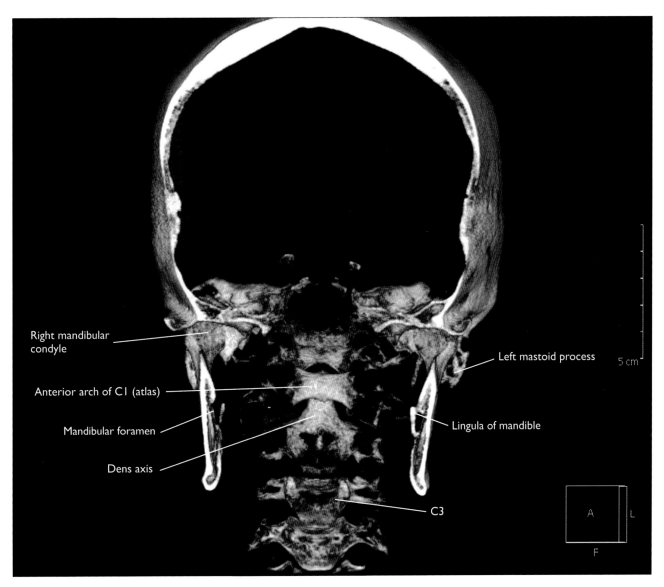

Right mandibular condyle

Anterior arch of C1 (atlas)

Mandibular foramen

Dens axis

Left mastoid process

Lingula of mandible

C3

5 cm

29

Fig 3-14 A 33.2-mm slice through the condyle.

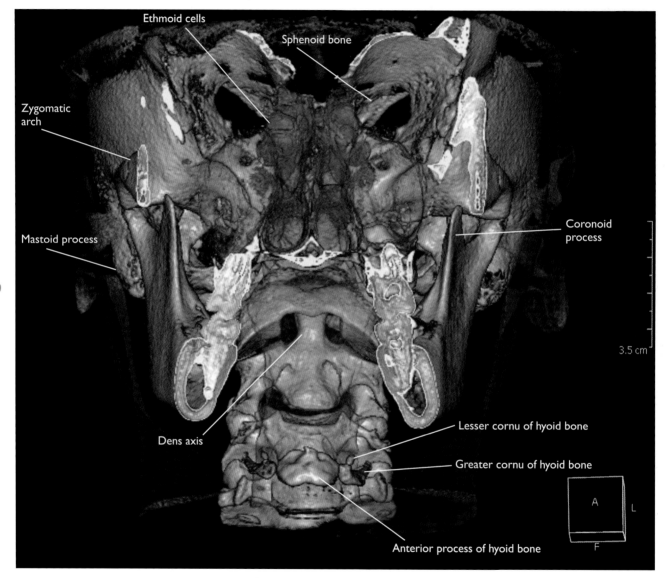

Fig 3-15 A 100-mm slice through the mandibular fossa showing the airway.

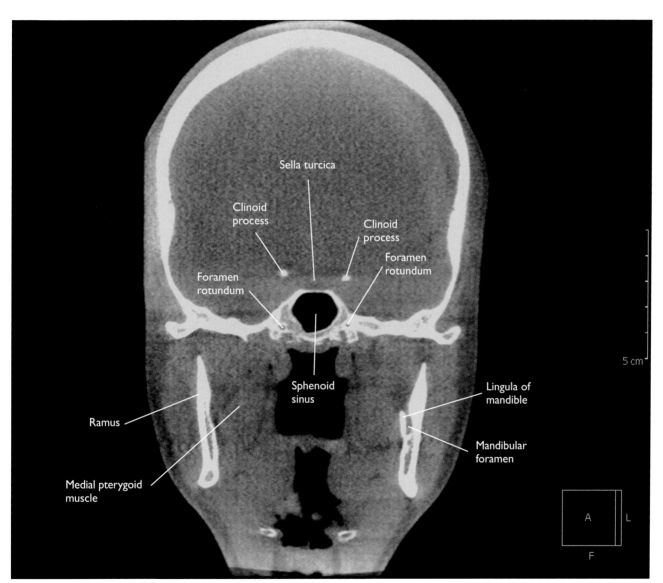

Sella turcica

Clinoid
process

Clinoid
process

Foramen
rotundum

Foramen
rotundum

Sphenoid
sinus

Lingula of
mandible

Ramus

Mandibular
foramen

Medial pterygoid
muscle

5 cm

A

L

F

Fig 3-16 A 0.15-mm slice through the middle of the sphenoid sinus.

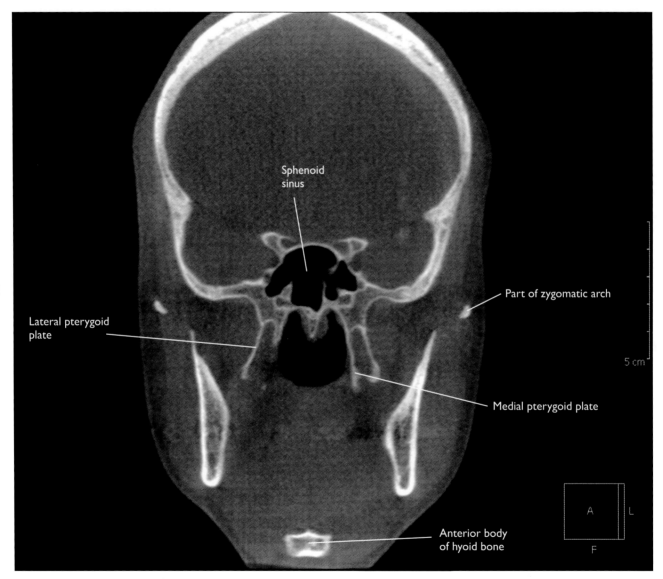

Fig 3-17 A 2-mm slice through the middle of the pterygoid plate.

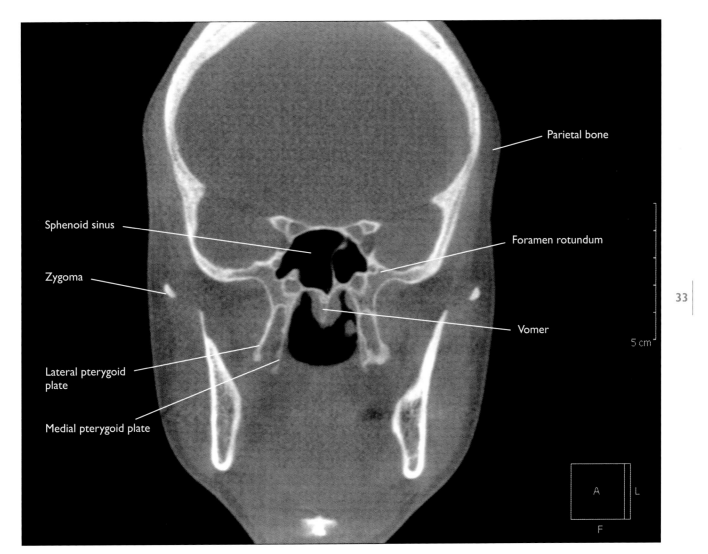

Parietal bone

Sphenoid sinus

Zygoma

Foramen rotundum

Lateral pterygoid
plate

Vomer

Medial pterygoid plate

5 cm

33

Fig 3-18 A closer view of a 0.15-mm slice through the middle of the pterygoid plates.

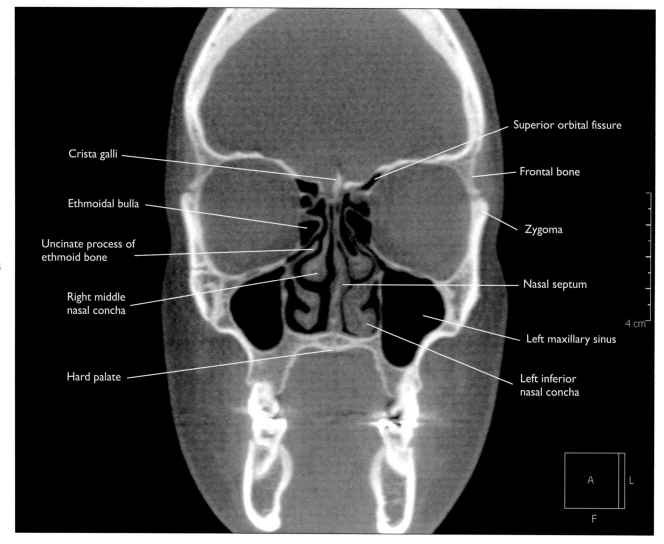

Crista galli

Ethmoidal bulla

Uncinate process of
ethmoid bone

Right middle
nasal concha

Hard palate

Superior orbital fissure

Frontal bone

Zygoma

Nasal septum

4 cm

Left maxillary sinus

Left inferior
nasal concha

34

Fig 3-19 A 0.15-mm slice through the posterior region of the maxillary sinus.

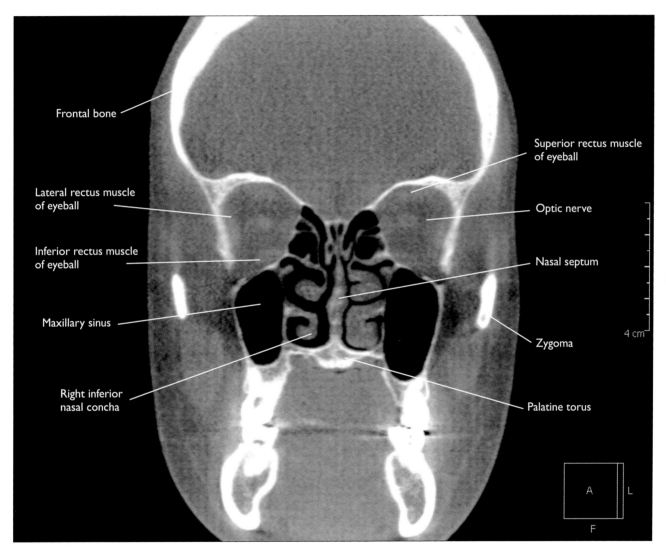

Frontal bone

Superior rectus muscle
of eyeball

Lateral rectus muscle
of eyeball

Optic nerve

Inferior rectus muscle
of eyeball

Nasal septum

Maxillary sinus

Zygoma

Right inferior
nasal concha

Palatine torus

4 cm

35

Fig 3-20 A 0.15-mm slice through the middle of the maxillary sinus.

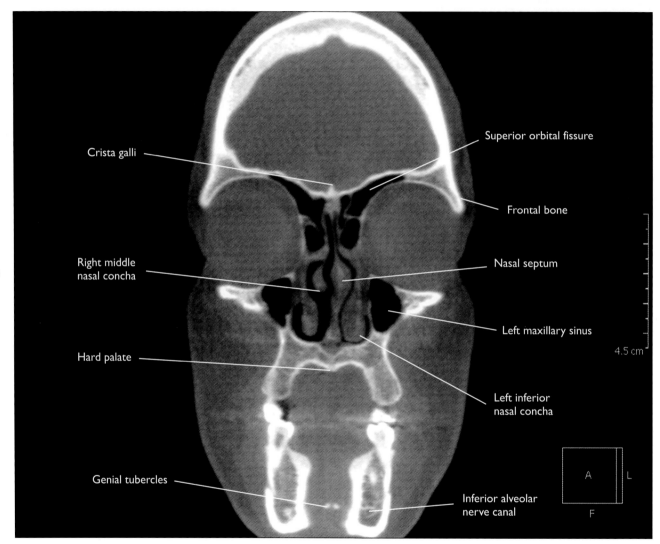

Fig 3-21 A 0.15-mm slice through the anterior region of the maxillary sinus.

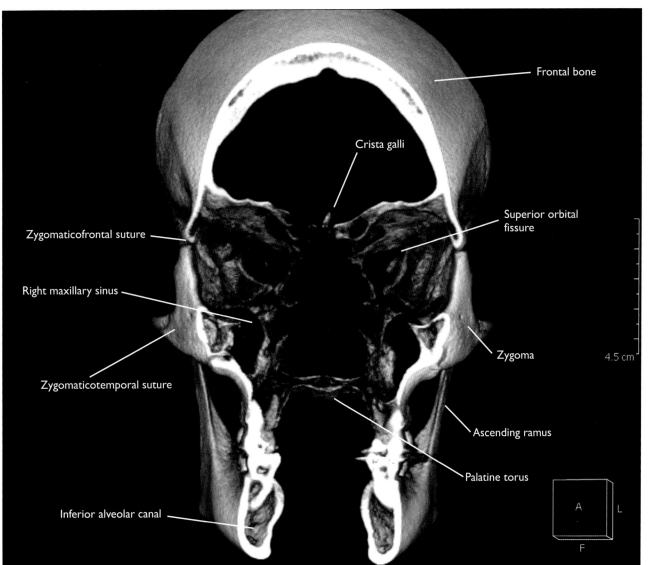

Fig 3-22 A 32.3-mm slice through the anterior region of the maxillary sinus.

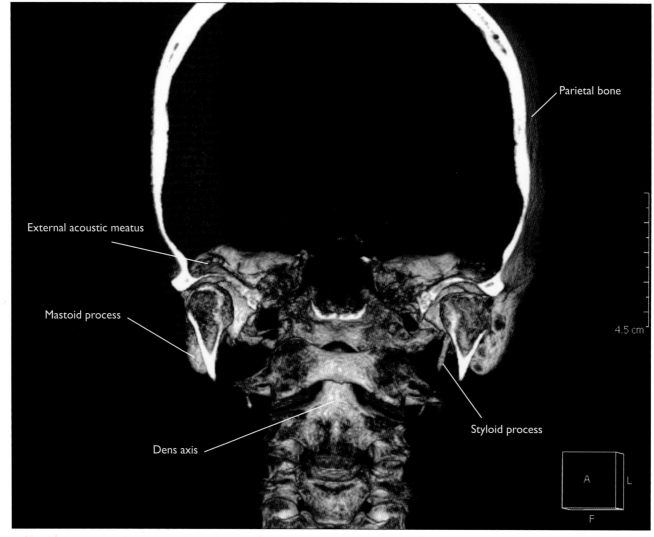

Parietal bone

External acoustic meatus

Mastoid process

Styloid process

Dens axis

4.5 cm

A

L

F

Fig 3-23 A 26.9-mm slice through the middle of the condyles.

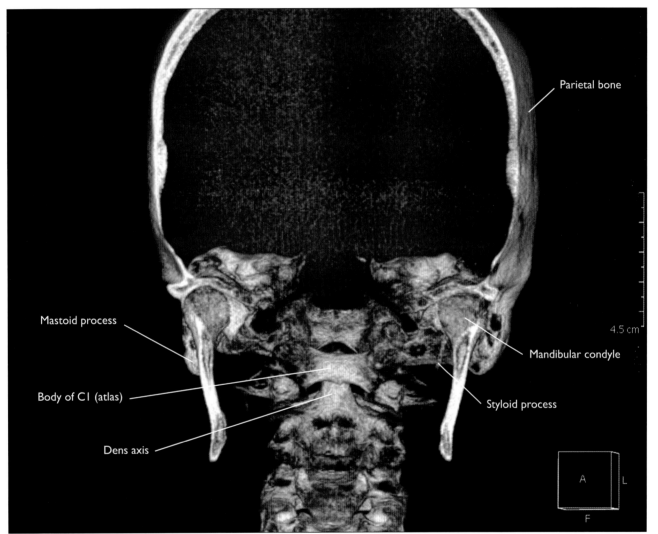

Parietal bone

Mastoid process

Mandibular condyle

Body of C1 (atlas)

Styloid process

Dens axis

4.5 cm

39

A | L

F

Fig 3-24 A 53.8-mm slice through the posterior region of the ramus.

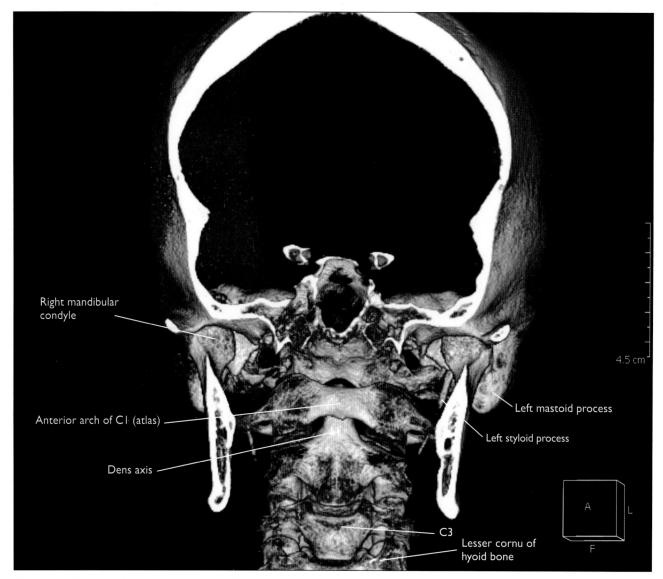

Right mandibular condyle

Anterior arch of C1 (atlas)

Dens axis

Left mastoid process

Left styloid process

C3

Lesser cornu of hyoid bone

4.5 cm

Fig 3-25 A 53.8-mm slice through the middle of the ascending ramus.

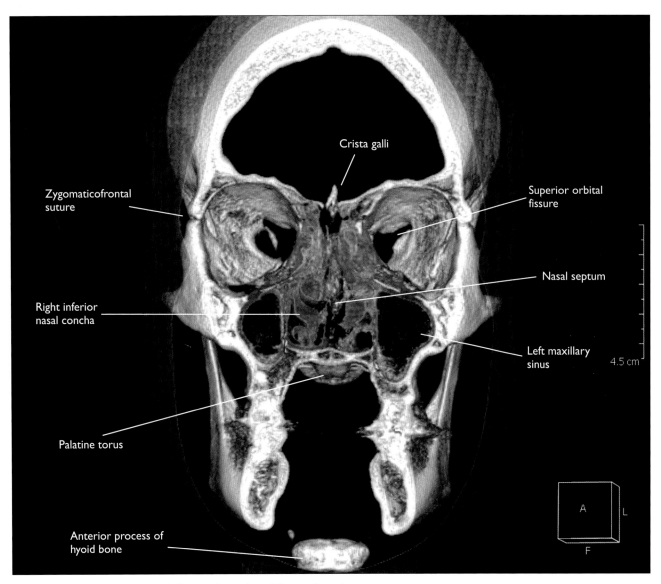

Crista galli

Zygomaticofrontal suture

Superior orbital fissure

Nasal septum

Right inferior nasal concha

Left maxillary sinus

4.5 cm

Palatine torus

Anterior process of hyoid bone

A

L

F

Fig 3-26 A 31.2-mm slice through the anterior region of the maxillary sinus.

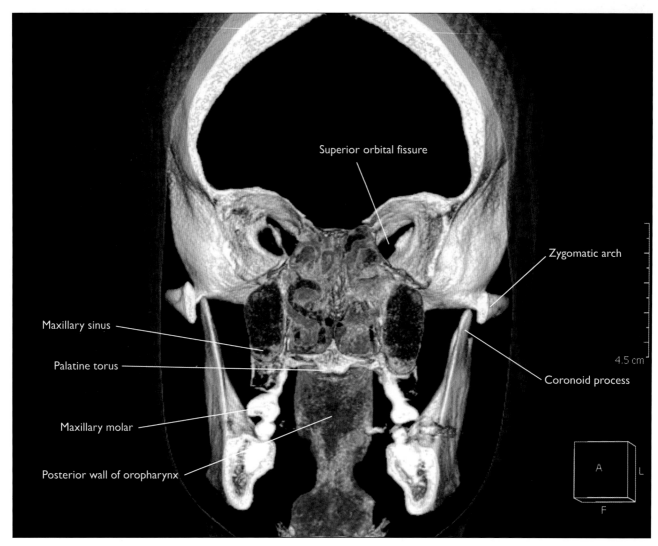

Superior orbital fissure

Zygomatic arch

4.5 cm

Coronoid process

Maxillary sinus

Palatine torus

Maxillary molar

Posterior wall of oropharynx

A

L

F

Fig 3-27 A 53.2-mm slice through the posterior region of the maxillary sinus.

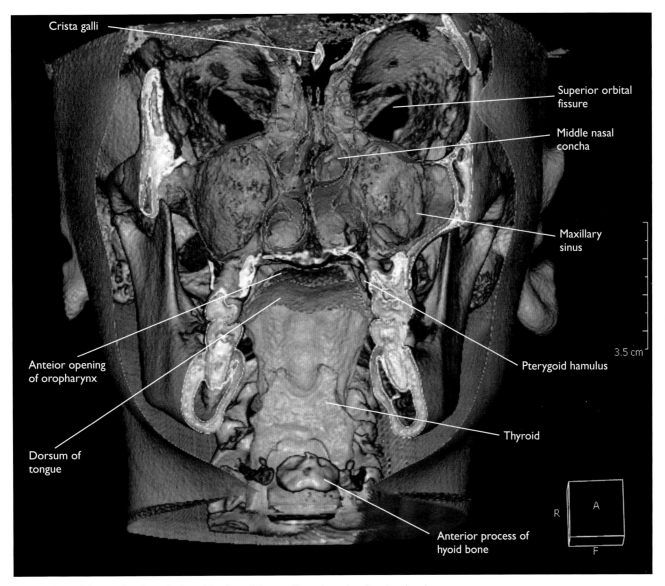

Crista galli

Superior orbital fissure

Middle nasal concha

Maxillary sinus

Pterygoid hamulus

Thyroid

Anterior process of hyoid bone

Dorsum of tongue

Anteior opening of oropharynx

3.5 cm

43

Fig 3-28 A 69.9-mm slice through the midregion of the maxillary sinus, also showing the airway.

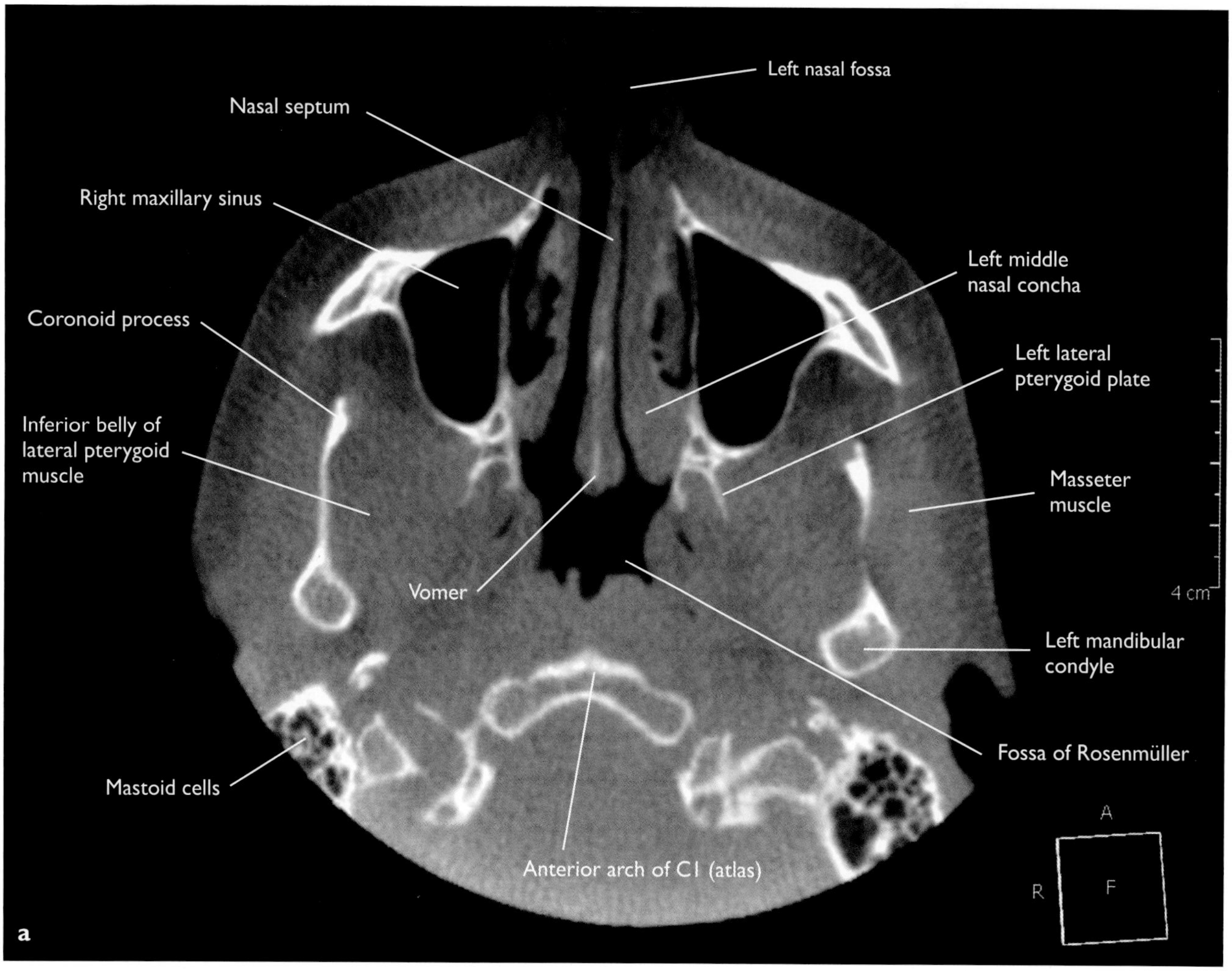

44

Left nasal fossa

Nasal septum

Right maxillary sinus

Left middle
nasal concha

Coronoid process

Left lateral
pterygoid plate

Inferior belly of
lateral pterygoid
muscle

Masseter
muscle

4 cm

Vomer

Left mandibular
condyle

Fossa of Rosenmüller

Mastoid cells

Anterior arch of C1 (atlas)

a

A

R F

Fig 3-29 Multiplanar reconstructed images showing (a) axial, (b) sagittal, and (c) coronal views through the midregion of the mandibular condyles.

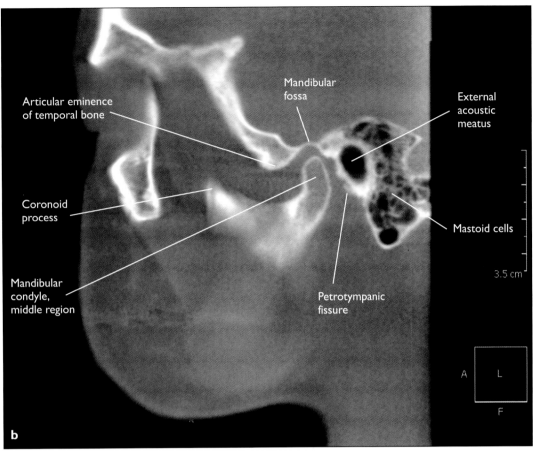

Articular eminence
of temporal bone

Coronoid
process

Mandibular
condyle,
middle region

Mandibular
fossa

External
acoustic
meatus

Mastoid cells

Petrotympanic
fissure

3.5 cm

A | L

F

b

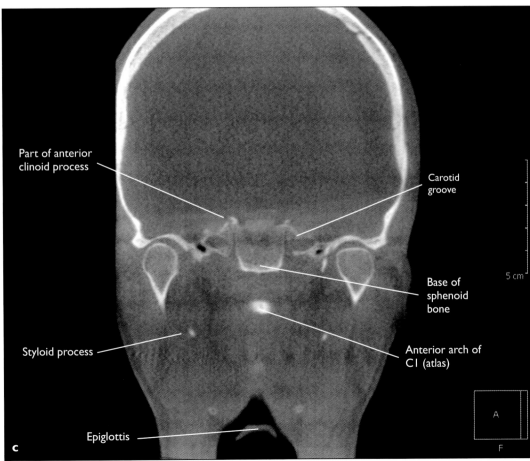

Part of anterior
clinoid process

Carotid
groove

Styloid process

Base of
sphenoid
bone

Anterior arch of
C1 (atlas)

5 cm

A

F

Epiglottis

c

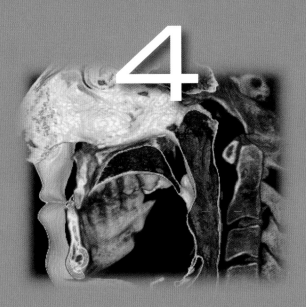

4

AIRWAY ANALYSIS

While a continuous positive airflow pressure (CPAP) appliance is still considered the first-line treatment for severe sleep apnea,[1] mild to moderate cases may be treated effectively with either a mandibular advancement device (MAD) or a tongue retraining device (TRD).[2] The MAD, which looks similar to a sports mouth guard and is the most common dental device for sleep apnea, directs the mandible forward and down slightly to keep the airway open during sleep. The TRD is a dental splint that holds the tongue in one place during sleep to keep the airway as open as possible.

Dentists who make appliances for patients experiencing sleep apnea have a significant role in the management of this disorder. The assessment of the patient's airway is an integral part of the management strategy. There appears to be no better way to visualize the airway than by employing cone beam volumetric imaging.

Fig

4-1

Airway Narrowing

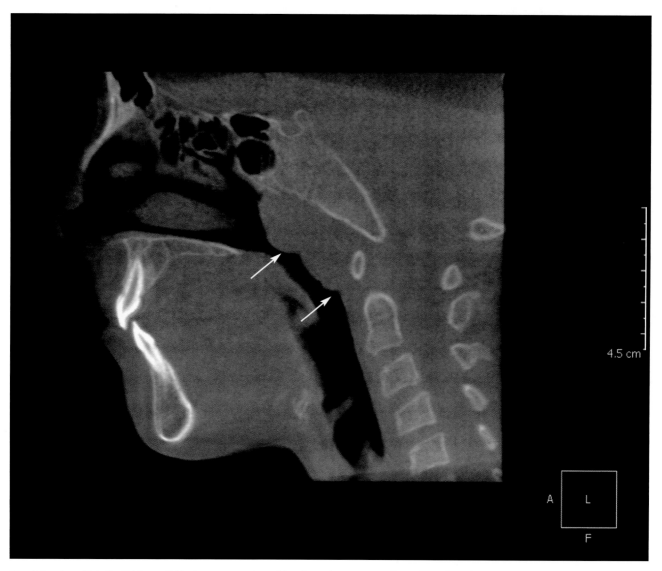

4.5 cm

Fig 4-1a A sagittal slice 0.15 mm thick shows narrowing of the airway in a young patient with enlarged adenoids *(arrows)*.

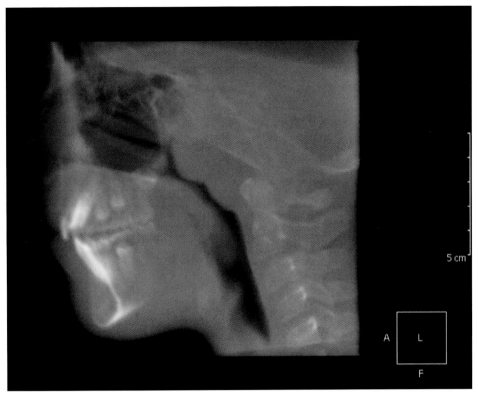

Fig 4-1b The airway is reconstructed in grayscale (40 mm thick) to resemble a typical cephalometric image.

49

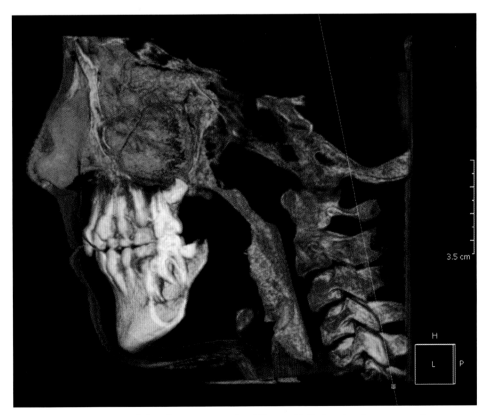

Fig 4-1c Sagittal image in 3-D color reconstruction (40 mm thick) showing airway narrowing.

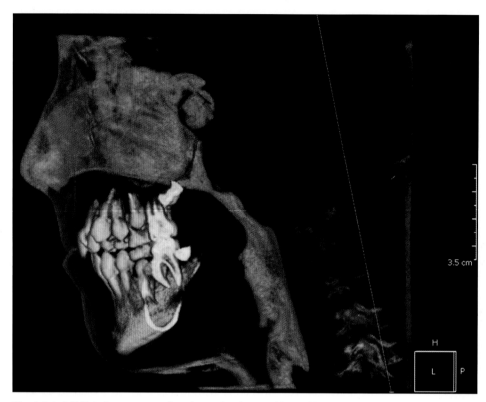

Fig 4-1d A 3-D color reconstruction shows the airway without the spinal column.

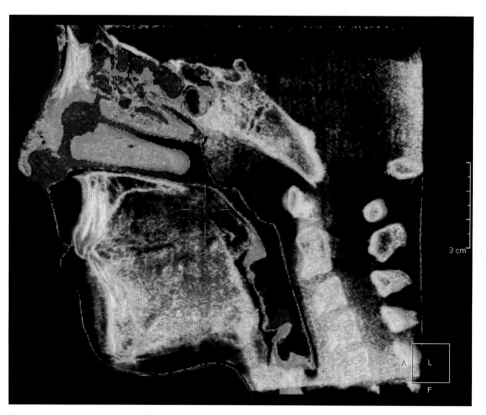

Fig 4-1e A slice only 5 mm thick shows the airway in 3-D color for assessment.

FIG

4-2

PATENT AIRWAY

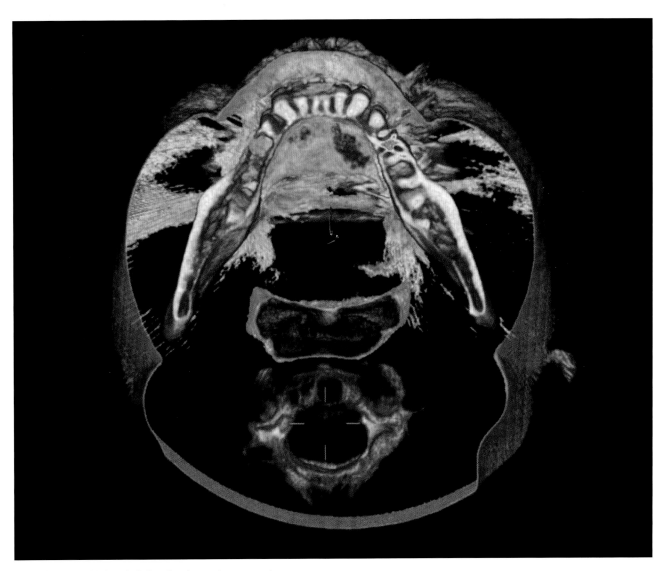

Fig 4-2a An axial view in 3-D color shows the patent airway space.

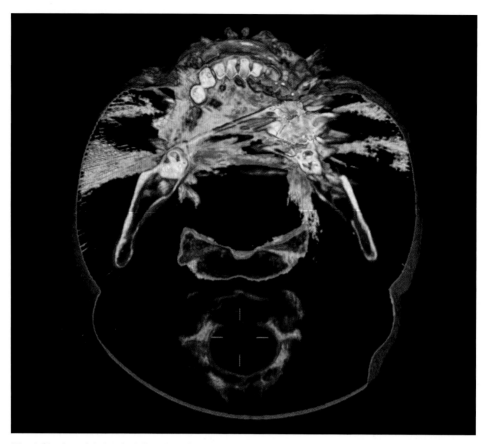

Fig 4-2b An axial view in 3-D color of the same patient shows the airway at the end of the uvula.

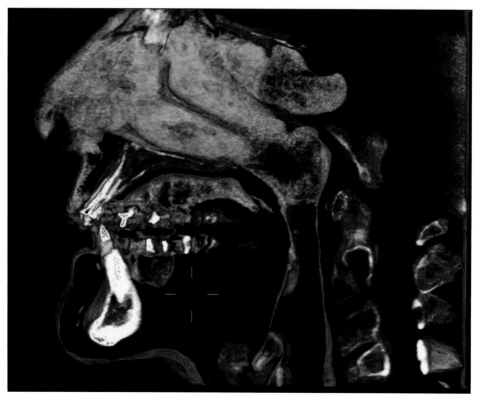

Fig 4-2c A 3-D color reconstruction of a sagittal slice 17.2 mm thick shows the airway (same patient as above). There is no restriction of the volume in this airway.

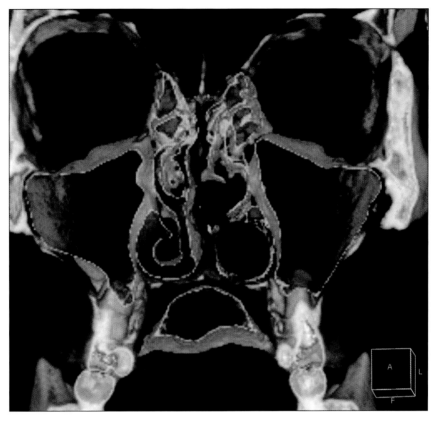

Fig 4-2d A coronal view of the same patient's airway in 3-D color is reconstructed in a slice 11.5 mm thick, representing the beginning of the nasopharyngeal airway. All other airway spaces such as the maxillary antra, nasal cavity, and ethmoid air cells also appear patent.

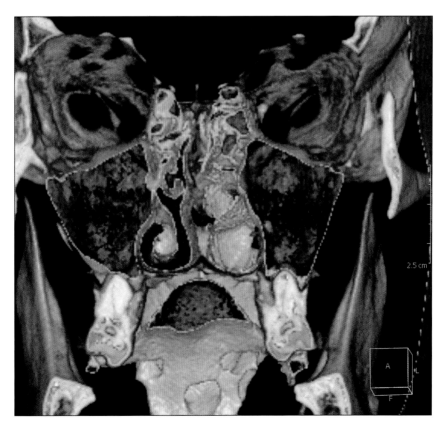

Fig 4-2e A 3-D color reconstruction of a coronal slice 30 mm thick of the same patient's airway represents the beginning of the nasopharyngeal airway. Note that the molars on each side of the maxillary arch are now visible.

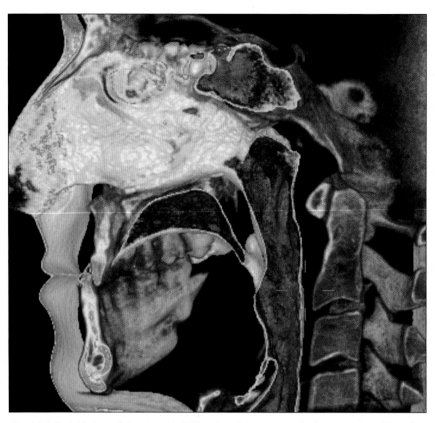

Fig 4-2f Sagittal view of the airway in 3-D color of the same patient, reconstructed in a slice 11.6 mm thick, representing the beginning of the nasopharyngeal airway. All other airway spaces such as the maxillary antra, nasal cavity, and ethmoid air cells also appear patent.

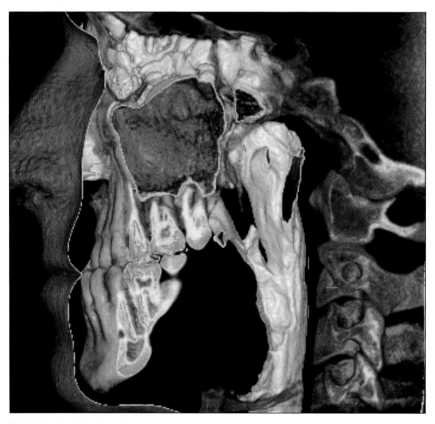

Fig 4-2g Sagittal view of the same patient's airway in 3-D color, reconstructed in a slice 30.1 mm thick. This represents the entire 3-D volume of the patient's airway.

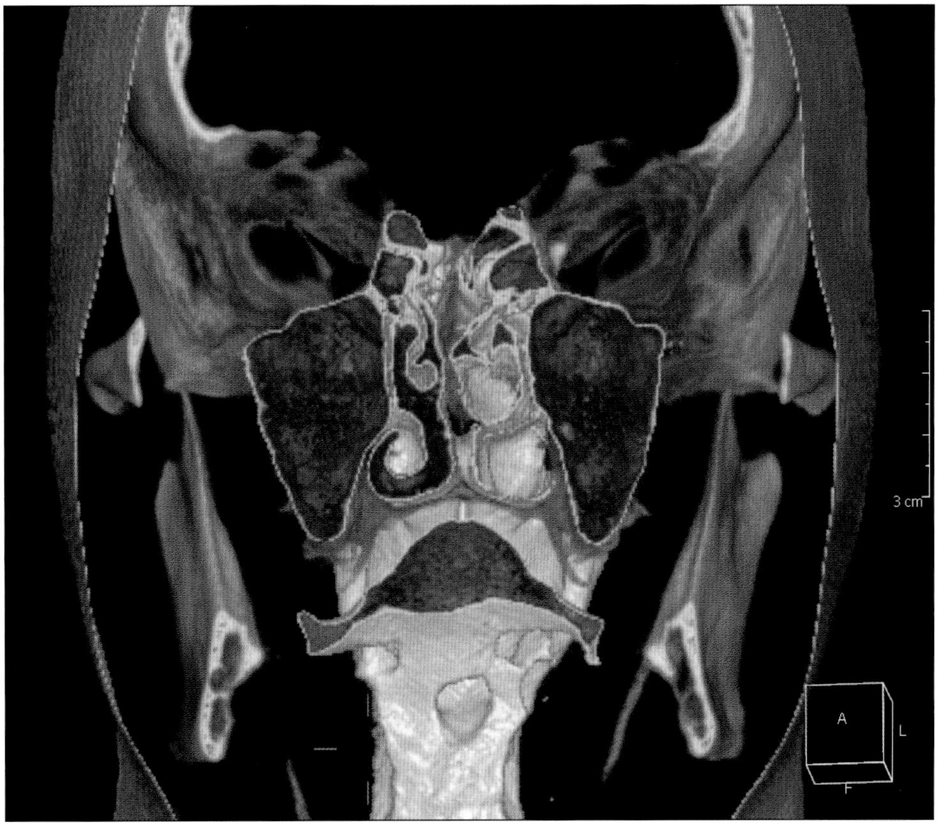

Fig 4-2h Same patient; this 3-D color reconstruction of an axial slice 30.1 mm thick shows the entire 3-D volume of the airway from the nasopharyngeal opening. Note also the patent maxillary sinuses.

REFERENCES

1. Bradley TD, Logan AG, Kimoff RJ, et al. Continuous positive airway pressure for central sleep apnea and heart failure. N Engl J Med 2005;353:2025–2033.

2. Kushida CA, Morgenthaler TI, Littner MR, et al. Practice parameters for the treatment of snoring and obstructive sleep apnea with oral appliances: An update for 2005. Sleep 2006;29:240–243.

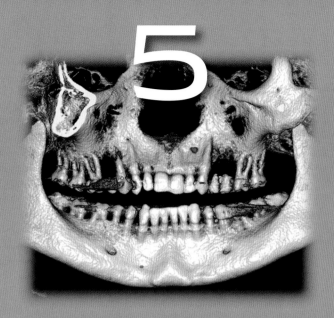

5

DENTAL FINDINGS

Even after patients undergo comprehensive clinical and radiographic examinations, their cone beam volumetric imaging data volumes referred for radiographic interpretation often reveal incidental dental findings; that is, dental diseases and conditions are found that could not be appreciated through plain film imaging alone. In some cases, even 2-D digital images (intraoral or panoramic) are insufficient to detect some dental lesions.

FIG
5-1

PERIAPICAL LESION

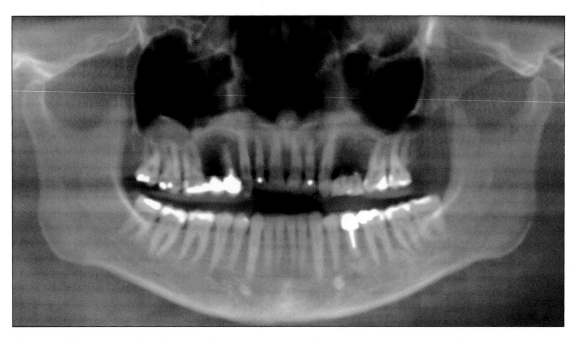

Fig 5-1a A 2-D reconstruction of a conventional panoramic image. The periapical lesion on the maxillary left canine is barely discernible and could be missed. Note also the mucous retention cyst in the right antrum.

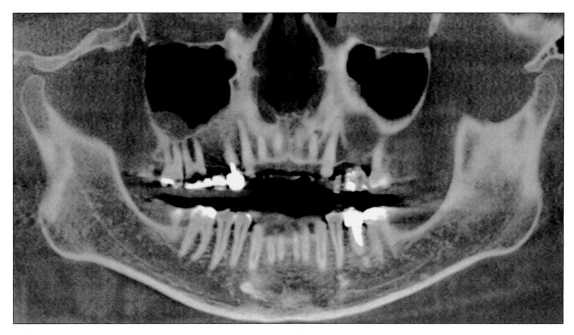

Fig 5-1b A thin slice (0.15 mm) 2-D pseudopanoramic image. The periapical lesion on the maxillary left canine is easily apparent in this thin section.

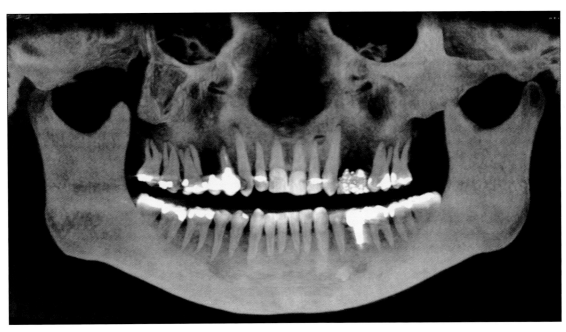

Fig 5-1c A 2-D maximum intensity projection (MIP) image of the same patient.

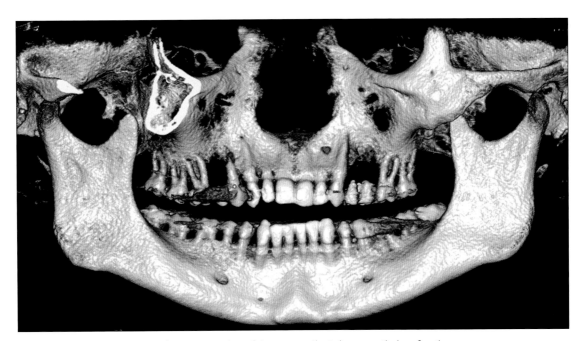

Fig 5-1d A 3-D color panoramic reconstruction of the same patient shows cortical perforation.

60

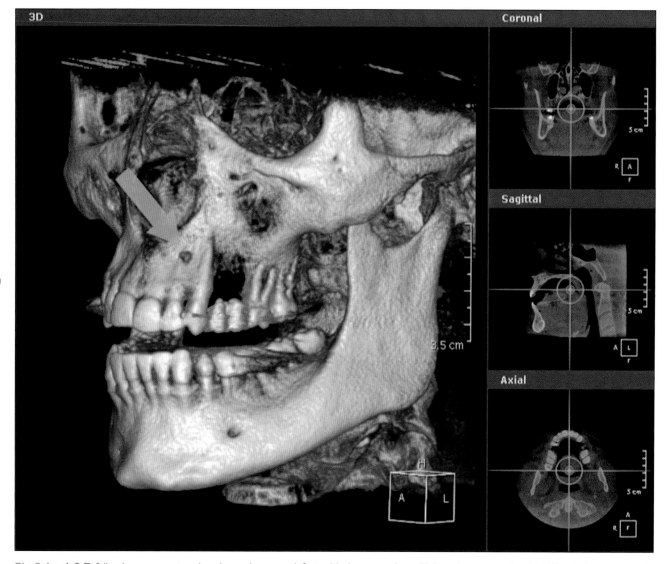

Fig 5-1e A 3-D full-volume reconstruction shows the same defect, with the grayscale multiplanar images on the right. The clinician can toggle between the images to completely visualize the lesion.

Fig

5-2

MESIODENS

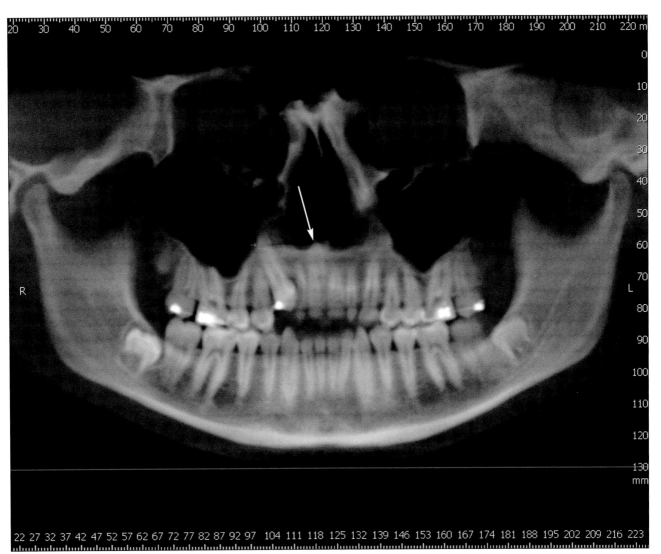

Fig 5-2a A conventional panoramic image. The mesiodens *(arrow)* was not very distinguishable.

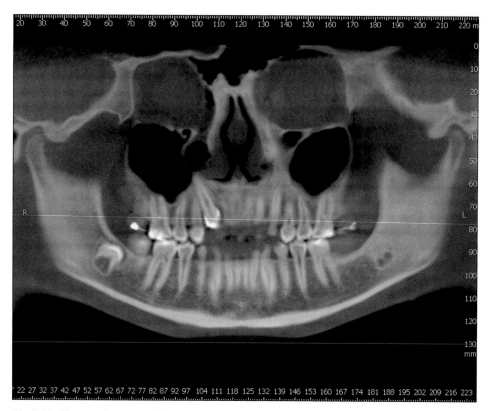

Fig 5-2b The pseudopanoramic image does not reveal the mesiodens, even in a thin slice.

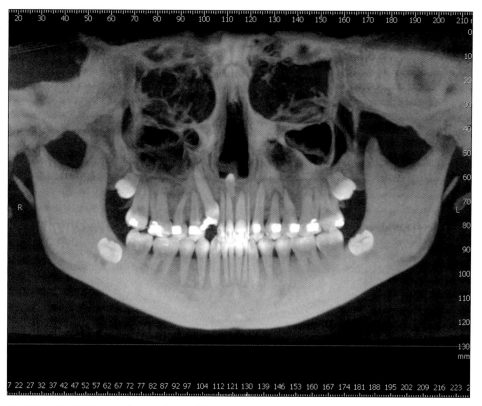

Fig 5-2c The MIP image, though distorted in the anterior region, shows the mesiodens easily.

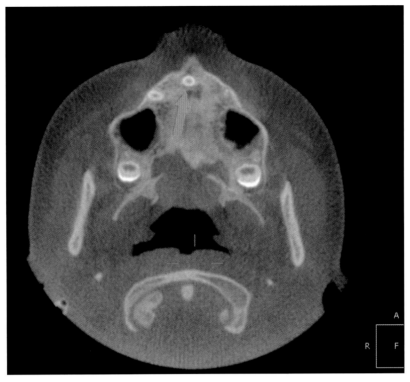

Fig 5-2d An axial slice shows the mesiodens *(arrow)* in relation to the beginning of the nasal cavity.

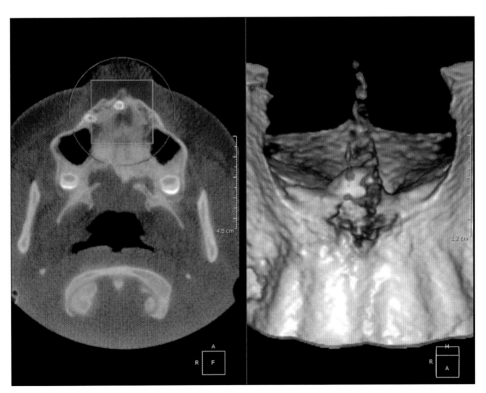

Fig 5-2e A 3-D reconstruction of the mesiodens area suggests eruption of the mesiodens into the right nasal cavity. This reconstruction is accomplished by using the Cube tool in the OnDemand 3D software (CyberMed International).

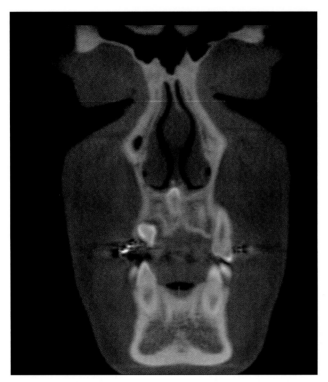

Fig 5-2f A 2-D grayscale coronal image with a partial view of the problem with the nasal cavity and mesiodens. The clinician would have to "stack" many slices to recognize the true extent of the lesion. In the 3-D color images from Figs 5-2e and 5-2g, the lesion is easily visualized.

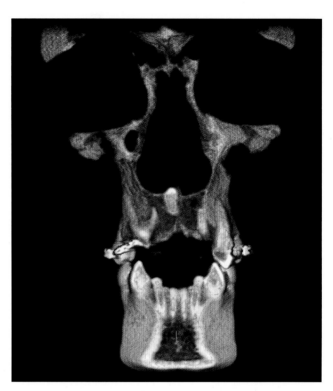

Fig 5-2g A 3-D slab (11.0 mm) rendering of the mesiodens from the coronal image in Fig 5-2f.

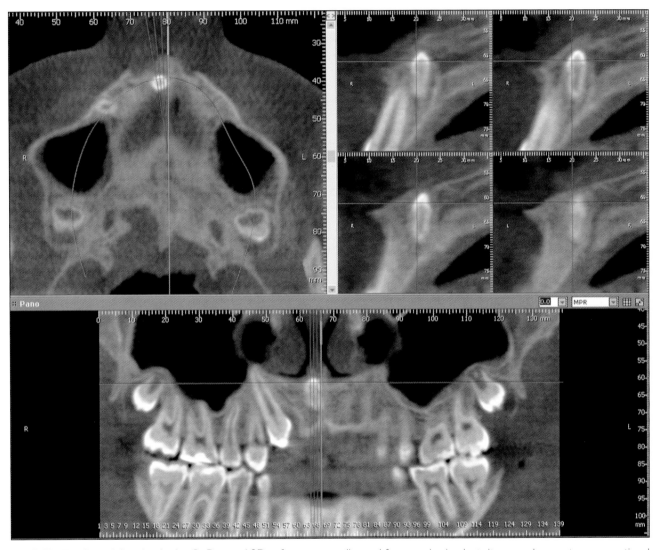

Fig 5-2h The Dental function in the OnDemand 3D software, normally used for assessing implant sites, can also create cross-sectional images of the mesiodens.

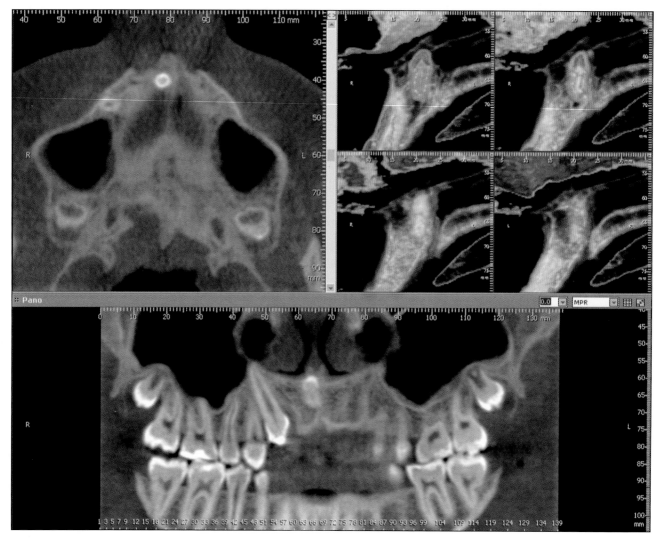

Fig 5-2i 3-D color rendering of selected images from Fig 5-2h shows the nasal cavity and maxillary sinus. Note that the thin layer of bone separating the mesiodens from the nasal cavity is more apparent in this reconstruction.

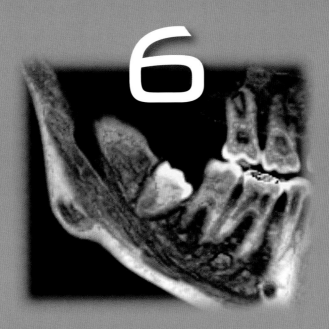

6

IMPACTED TEETH

Impacted teeth are a common problem. Orthodontists and oral and maxillofacial surgeons spend a lot of time assessing tooth position and eruption patterns and managing patients referred from general dentists who have usually seen these impactions on intraoral or panoramic radiographs. Permanent canines erupting abnormally are common, as are horizontally impacted mandibular third molars. Even supernumerary teeth are a common enough anomaly to require additional radiographic assessment. Cone beam volumetric imaging (CBVI) is the most appropriate way to perform this assessment for preoperative planning and orthodontic management. It is likely that CBVI will become the standard of care for the assessment of all impactions in the near future.

FIG

6-1

MAXILLARY CANINE AND MANDIBULAR THIRD MOLAR

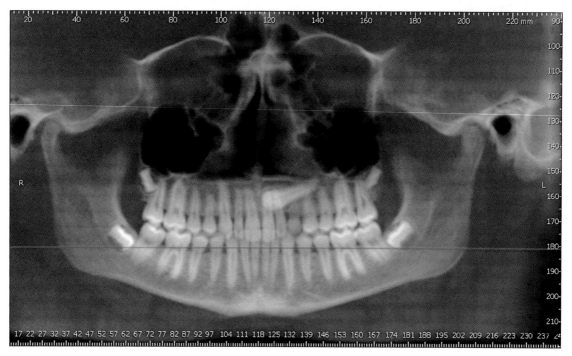

Fig 6-1a A panoramic image, reconstructed from the cone beam data volume, represents the type of image that would serve for the initial assessment of the missing canine. There is no way to determine the correct orientation (facial or palatal position) from this panoramic image. The primary canine is retained. The permanent canine is impacted horizontally.

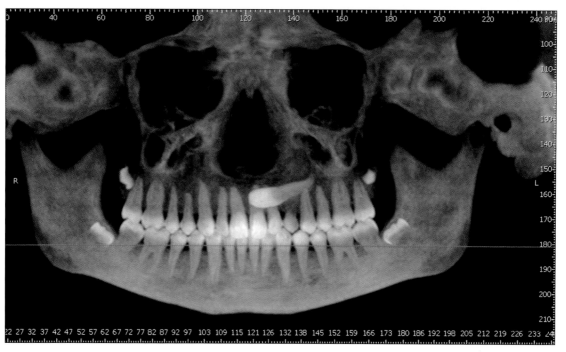

Fig 6-1b The same image as Fig 6-1a, using a maximum intensity projection view. The canine appears to be anterior to the central and lateral incisors.

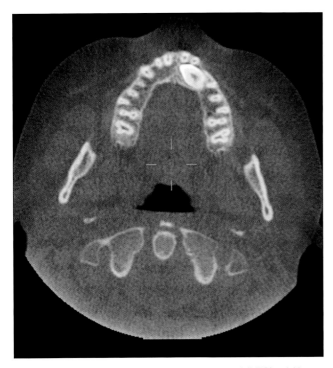

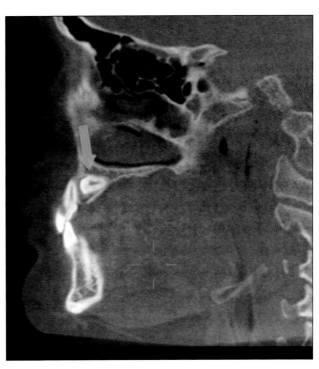

Fig 6-1c The cone beam multiplanar reconstructed (MPR) axial image reveals the correct position of this impacted canine. It is posterior to the central and lateral incisors and the retained primary canine.

Fig 6-1d The cone beam MPR sagittal image reveals the position of this impacted canine *(arrow)* relative to the left lateral incisor.

Fig 6-1e The cone beam MPR coronal image reveals the position of this impacted canine as posterior to the central and lateral incisors.

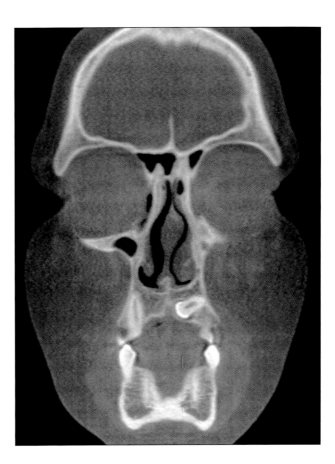

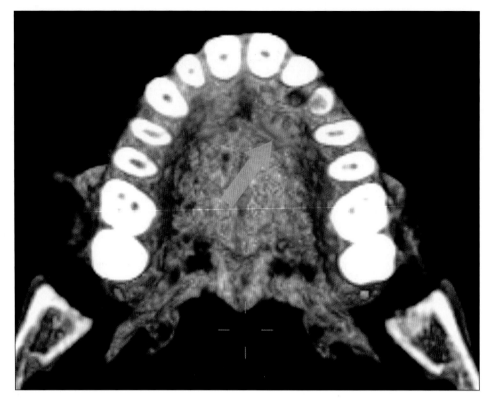

Fig 6-1f A 3-D color reconstruction shows the palatal elevation caused by the impacted canine *(arrow)*.

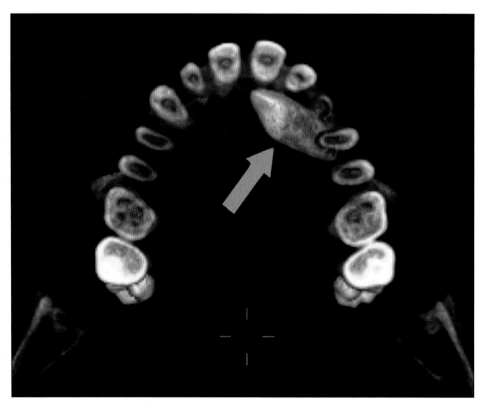

Fig 6-1g A 3-D color reconstruction (18.3 mm thick) shows the canine position *(arrow)* unobstructed by bony anatomy.

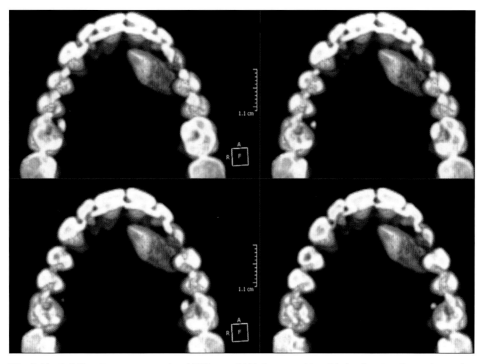

Fig 6-1h A 3-D color reconstruction (18.3 mm thick) formatted in a "4-view" series shows the canine position unobstructed by bony anatomy at the level of the incisal edges of the maxillary and mandibular anterior teeth.

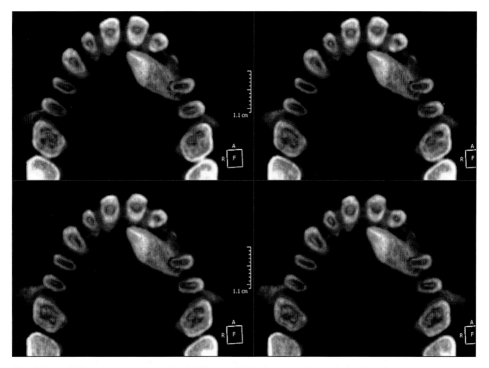

Fig 6-1i A 3-D color reconstruction (18.3 mm thick) formatted in a "4-view" series shows the canine position unobstructed by bony anatomy at the level of the midregion of the pulp canals of the maxillary premolars.

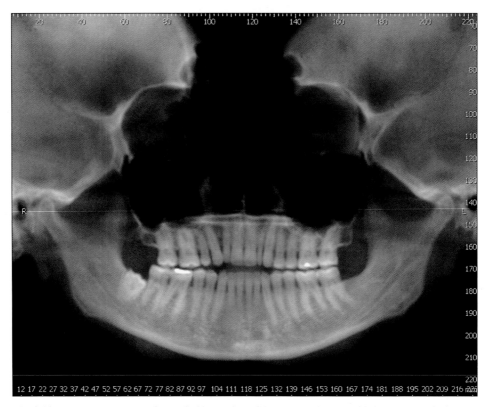

Fig 6-1j A panoramic image of a vertical impaction of the mandibular right third molar reveals that the inferior alveolar nerve canal passes close to the apex.

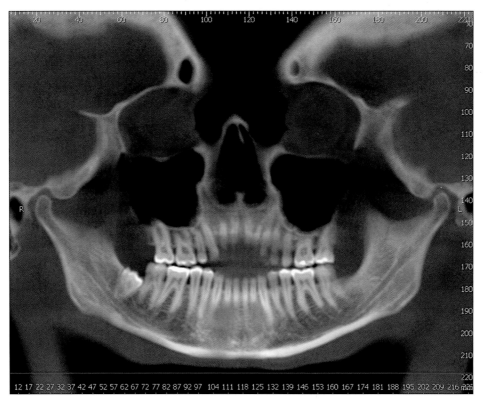

Fig 6-1k A pseudopanoramic image (5.0 mm) provides a sharper view of the vertical impaction of the mandibular right third molar. The inferior alveolar nerve canal now appears to touch the apex of the tooth.

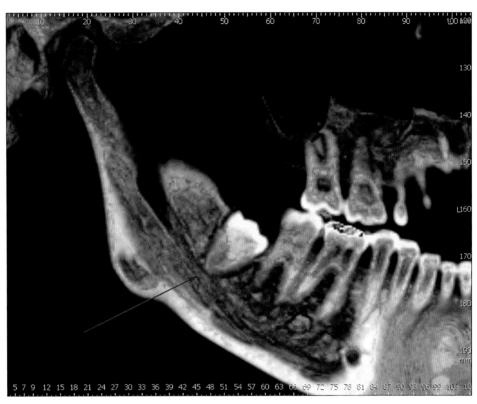

Fig 6-11 A 3-D reconstructed view of the region shows a vertical impaction of the mandibular right third molar, with the inferior alveolar nerve touching the apex of the tooth *(arrow)*.

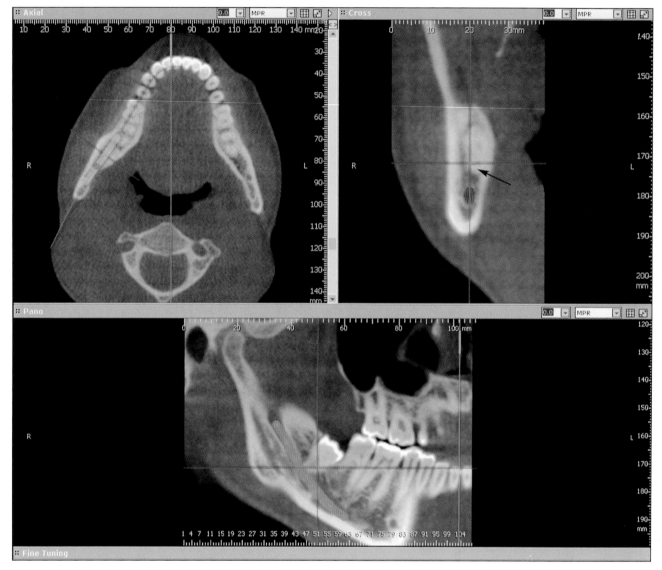

Fig 6-1m Axial, sagittal, and pseudopanoramic images with the nerve canal drawn in and a reference line at the midroot level. At this location, the cross-sectional image *(top right)* reveals that the inferior alveolar nerve *(red oval)* does *not* touch the mandibular third molar *(arrow)*.

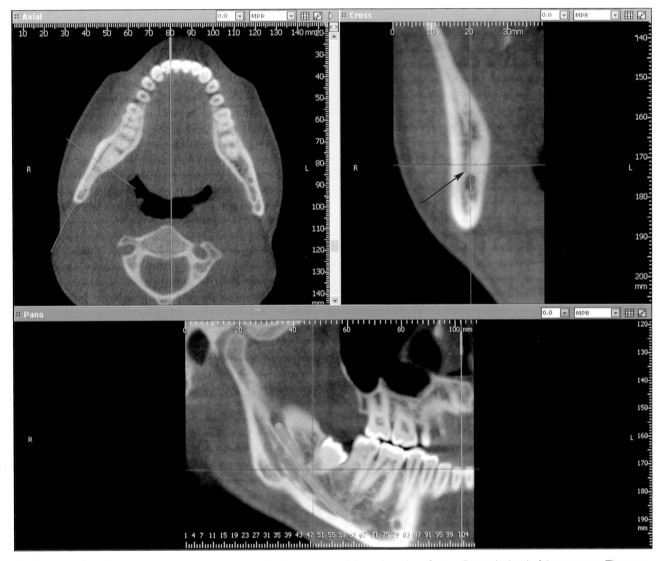

Fig 6-1n Axial, sagittal, and pseudopanoramic images with the nerve canal drawn in and a reference line at the level of the root apex. The cross-sectional image *(top right)* reveals that the inferior alveolar nerve *(red oval) does* touch the apex of the mandibular third molar *(arrow)*.

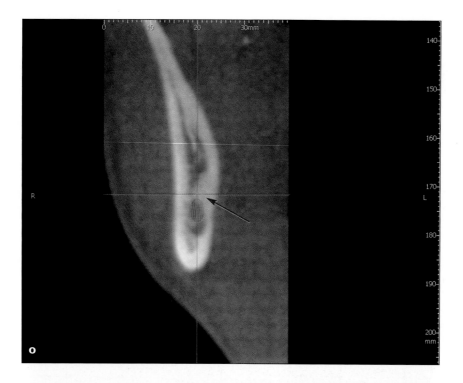

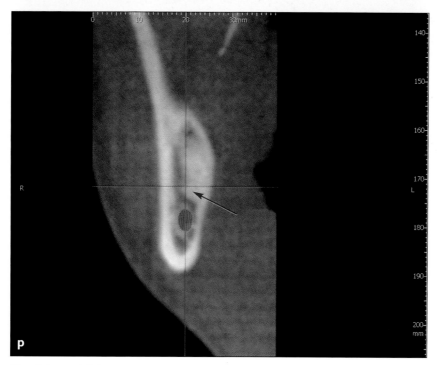

Figs 6-1o and 6-1p Cross-sectional images with a reference line at the root apex region confirm that the inferior alveolar nerve *(red ovals) does* touch the very apex of the tooth *(arrows)*.

FIG
6-2

MAXILLARY THIRD MOLARS

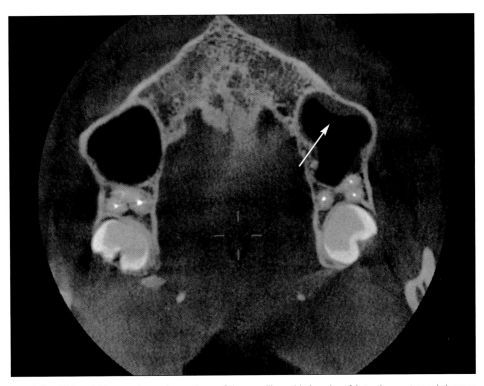

Fig 6-2a This axial image shows impactions of the maxillary third molars. Note the root canal therapy on the second molars, as well as some minor mucosal thickening in the left maxillary sinus *(arrow)*.

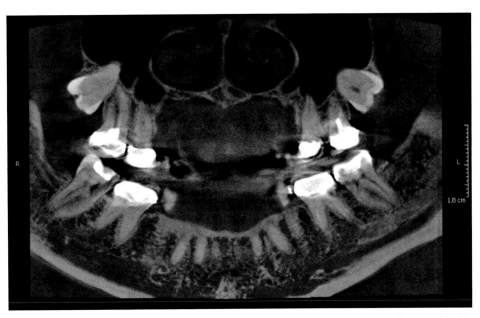

Fig 6-2b A pseudopanoramic image (0.16 mm thick) shows the impactions seen in Fig 6-2a. This thin section is not in the correct plane to show the maxillary anterior teeth; however, these could be imaged by scrolling anteriorly through the arch to the appropriate plane of section.

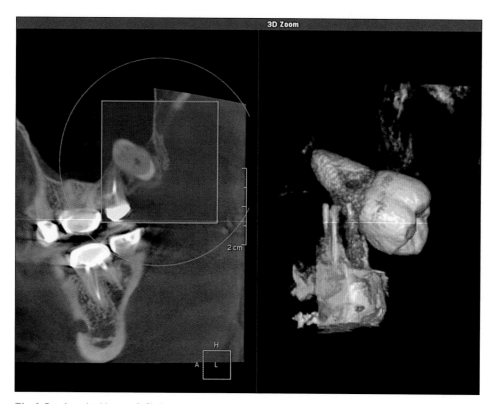

Fig 6-2c A sagittal image *(left)* shows impaction of the maxillary left third molar; the Cube tool *(right)* is used to render the 3-D image of the maxillary second and third molars. Note the detail of the occlusal surface. This is a small-volume image taken using the ProMax 3D machine (Planmeca) and imaged with N-Liten 3D software (Planmeca).

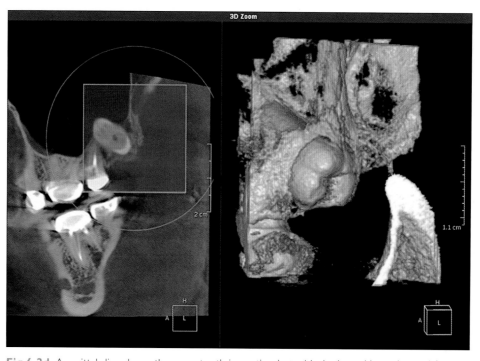

Fig 6-2d A sagittal slice shows the same tooth impaction but with the buccal bone imaged for preoperative evaluation. Detailed anatomy is again visualized. This image was reconstructed using the ProMax 3D machine and N-Liten 3D software.

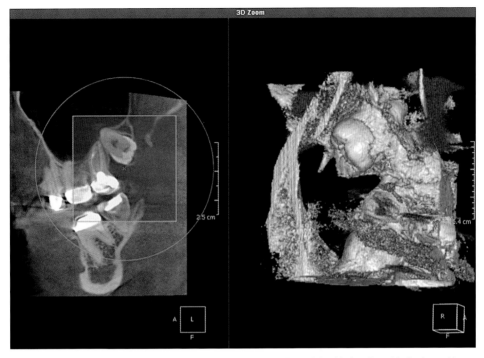

Fig 6-2e This sagittal image shows the impaction of the maxillary right third molar with the buccal bone imaged for preoperative evaluation. The maxillary sinus is colored violet. This image was reconstructed using the ProMax 3D machine and N-Liten 3D software.

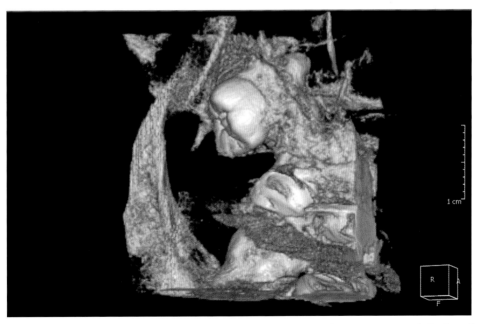

Fig 6-2f A 3-D color rendering shows the same impaction as in Fig 6-2e without extra colorization of air space.

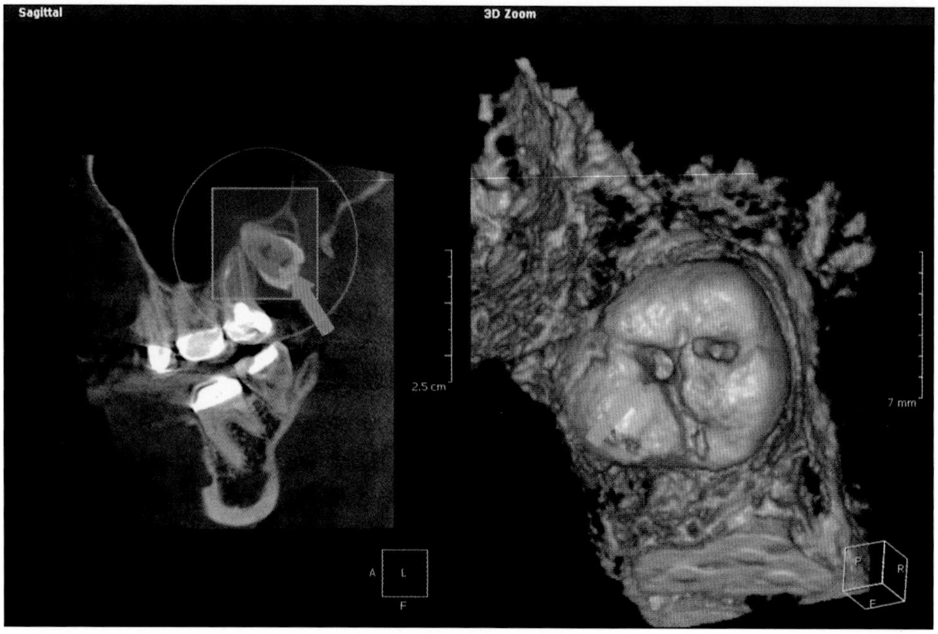

Fig 6-2g The image area from Fig 6-2f is rendered in 3-D and color, and rotated to show the occlusal surface of the tooth *(right)*. Because of the communication of this tooth with the oral cavity, these pit depressions *(arrow)* may be caries lesions. Image rendered using the ProMax 3D machine and N-Liten 3D software.

7

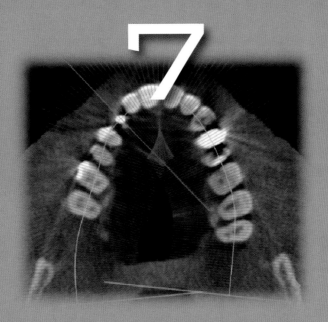

IMPLANT SITE ASSESSMENT

Probably the most common use for cone beam volumetric imaging (CBVI), after orthodontic evaluation, is preoperative implant site assessment. When a clinician is placing multiple implants for an overdenture, use of CBVI for site assessment is indispensable. However, cases involving multiple implants and horizontal anchorage of the surgical guide are not nearly as common as cases involving single tooth loss. With the precision of CBVI, any clinician wishing to perform surgery for an implant or restorative procedure can easily work on preoperative planning without referring all surgical procedures to a specialist. The illustrated cases are not intended to establish protocol for single implant site assessment, but rather demonstrate the precision with which measurement and location can be performed using appropriate CBVI software.

IMPORTANCE OF A RADIOGRAPHIC STENT AND MARKER

The importance of using a radiographic stent with a non-metallic marker for implant site location cannot be overstated. Radiographic stents, which help to precisely locate the desired bone receptor site, have been around for many years.[1] The clinician provides the history, casts, and clinical findings (including preliminary 2-D radiographic information) and is the operator who places or directs the placement of the implant. Providing a stent and a precise description of the most desirable location is essential to allow the radiologist and/or technician to take precise measurements of length, width, and angulation for the implant site. If the clinician is analyzing the site, a marker will invariably assist the evaluation. Placing a radiopaque marker at the clinically determined location makes all subsequent steps much easier.

Software is available to perform measurements to within about 0.1 mm. These measurements are ideally performed at the site indicated by the radiographic marker. *Metal markers and barium pastes should not be used because of the inevitable artifacts and image degradation.* Metallic balls such as copper balls may be suitable, but gutta-percha is probably the ideal marker material. An article describing the simple construction of a radiographic stent is available at the LearnDigital website.[2]

FIG

7-1

CREATING A RADIOGRAPHIC STENT

Fig 7-1a A clinical cast is shown in a surveyor with a coffee stir stick as stylus. Guttapercha will be placed into one half of the stick to provide a radiopaque marker that will not produce scatter artifacts in the volume data.

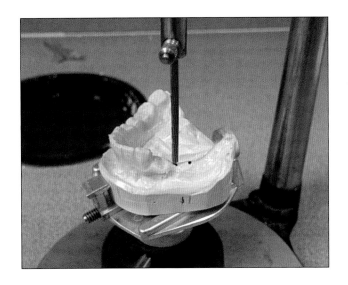

Fig 7-1b The clinical cast is shown with the processed acrylic stent and coffee stir stick with gutta-percha inside. A hot-wax instrument is then used to cut off the excess gutta-percha, and the marker area is covered with new cold-cure acrylic. Retention is provided during image acquisition by the incisal/occlusal imprint. (Fig 7-1 courtesy of Dr Ron Shelley, Glendale, AZ.)

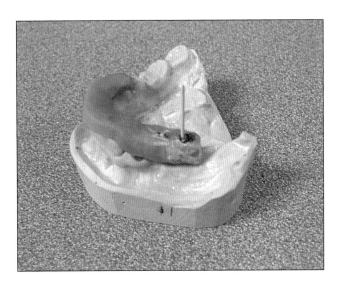

FIG

7-2

CANINE SITE ASSESSMENT

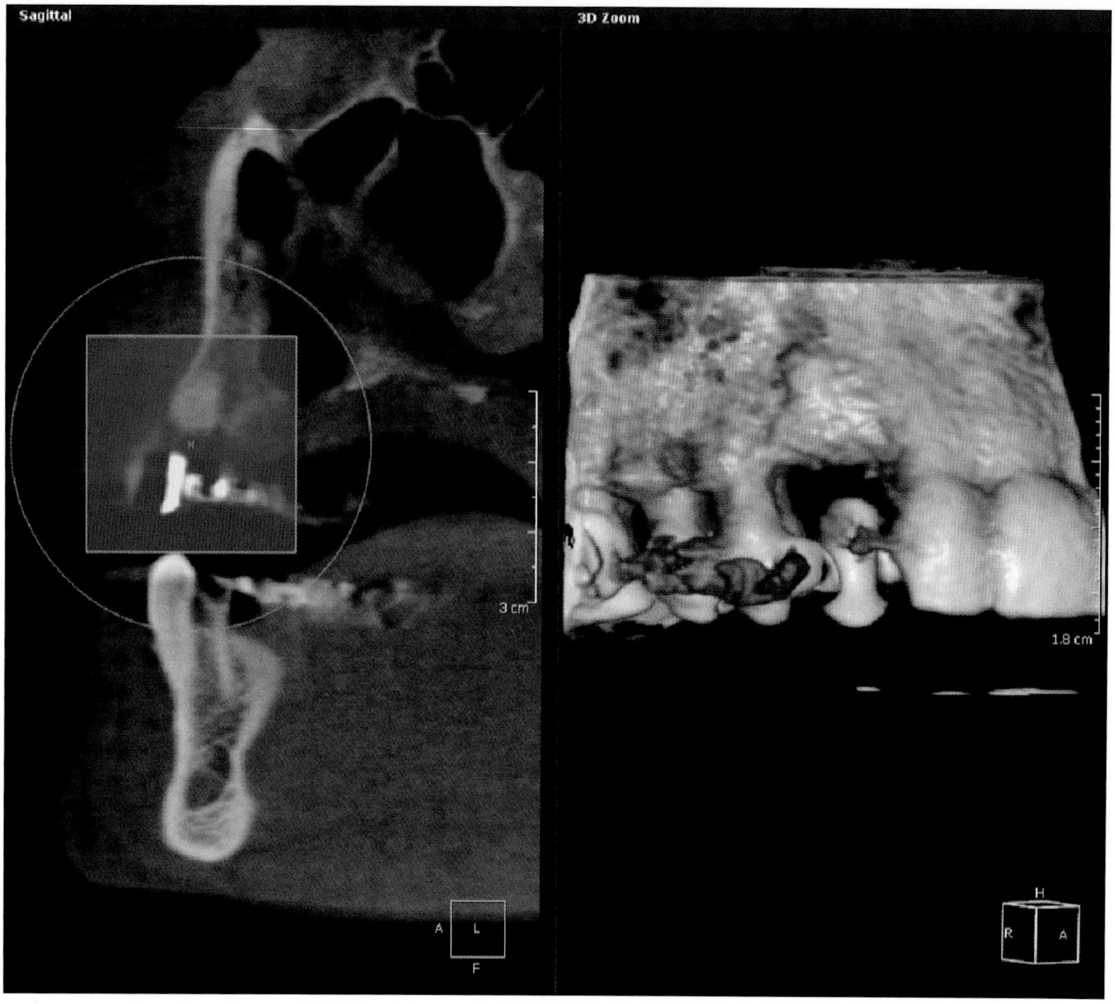

Fig 7-2a A sagittal view *(left)* and a 3-D color reconstruction *(right)* show the metallic marker used to locate the ideal implant site.

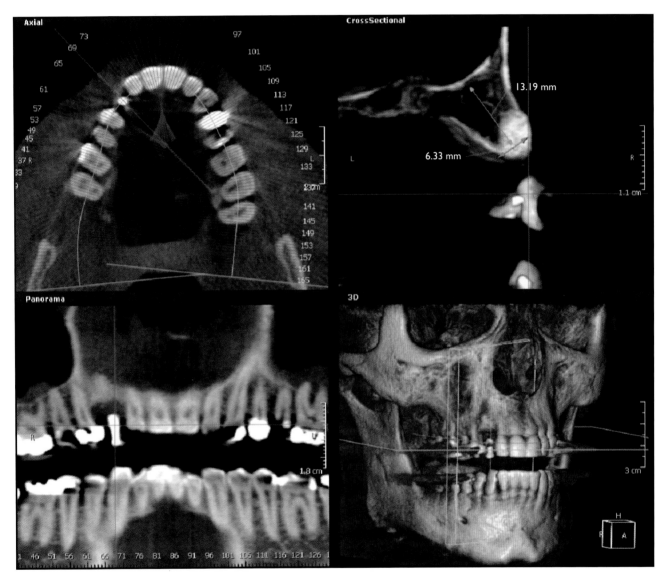

Fig 7-2b With a marker in the implant site, the length, width, and even angulation can be measured precisely in preparation for implant selection.

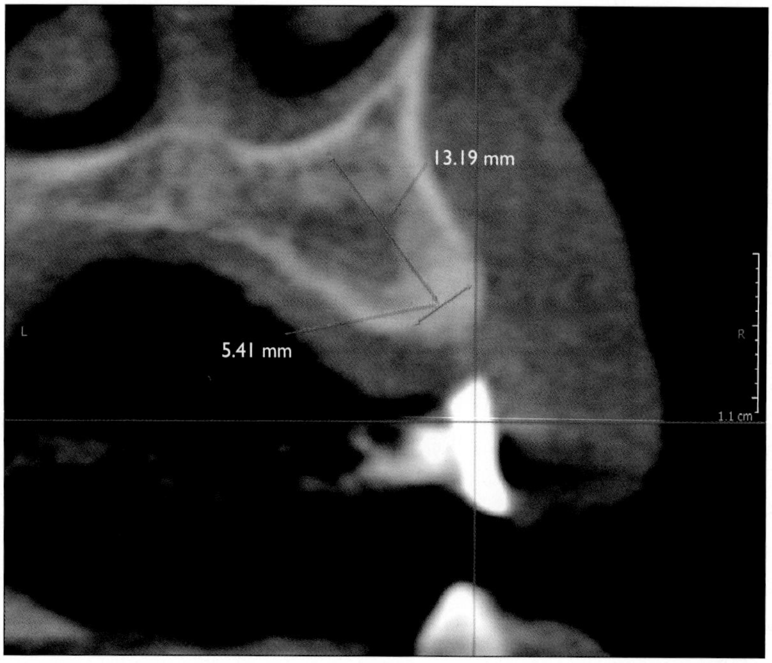

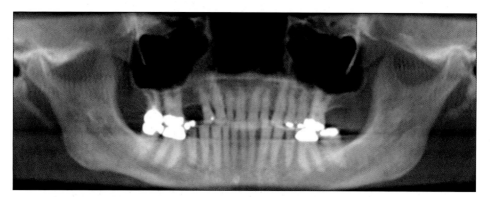

13.19 mm

5.41 mm

L

R

1.1 cm

Fig 7-2c A close-up of the proposed implant site shows the ridge width and bone height within one-tenth of a millimeter.

FIG
7-3

PREMOLAR SITE ASSESSMENT

Fig 7-3a Panoramic image of proposed implant site for the maxillary right second premolar. With this type of 2-D image it is *not* possible to measure the precise distance to the maxillary sinus or the width of the alveolar bone from the facial wall to the palatal wall.

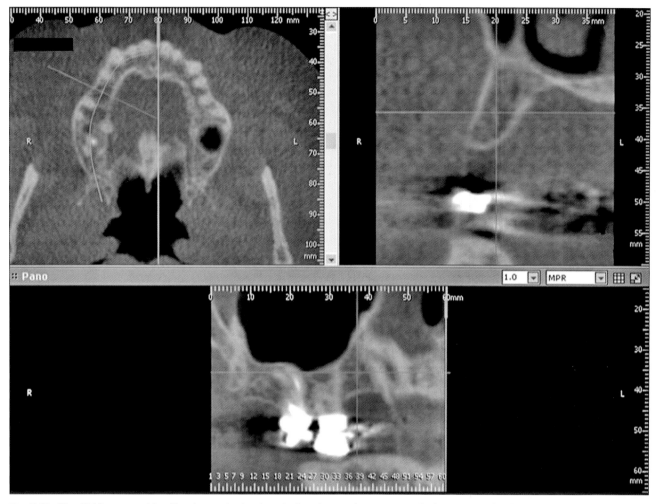

Fig 7-3b The CBVI program identifies the precise implant site location, ready to measure, in the cross-sectional view.

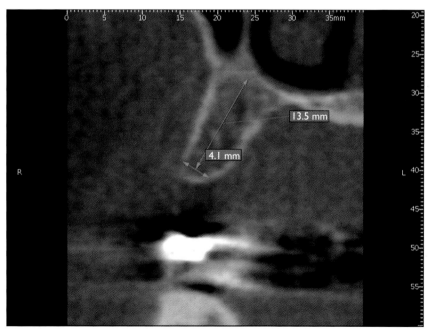

Fig 7-3c The CBVI program shows the measurement of the implant site in the cross-sectional view.

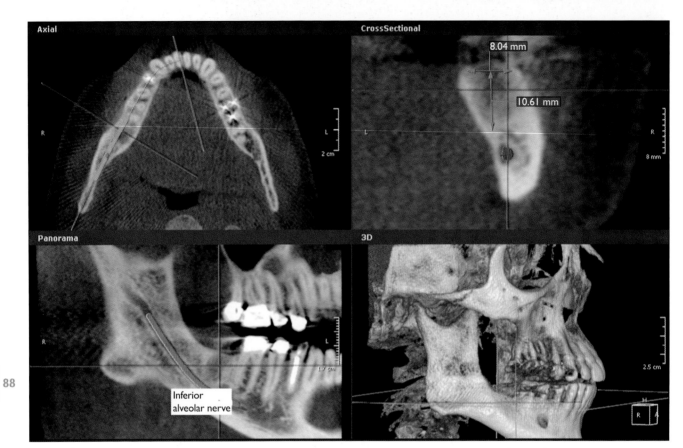

FIG

7-4

MOLAR SITE ASSESSMENT

Fig 7-4a The CBVI program shows the precise location of the inferior alveolar nerve, as well as the reference line at the proposed implant site location. The nerve canal has been automatically labeled in red after the arch and canal have been drawn using the simple program tools.

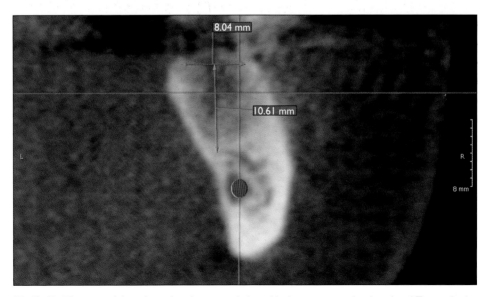

Fig 7-4b Close-up of the selected and measured site with the nerve canal colored red. To stay in the center of the alveolar ridge and engage the cortical bone, an implant measuring 4.5 mm × 10 mm may be used safely. Implant selection based on 2-D panoramic imaging alone would have resulted in a longer implant and possible perforation into the submandibular fossa because of height distortion in the radiograph.

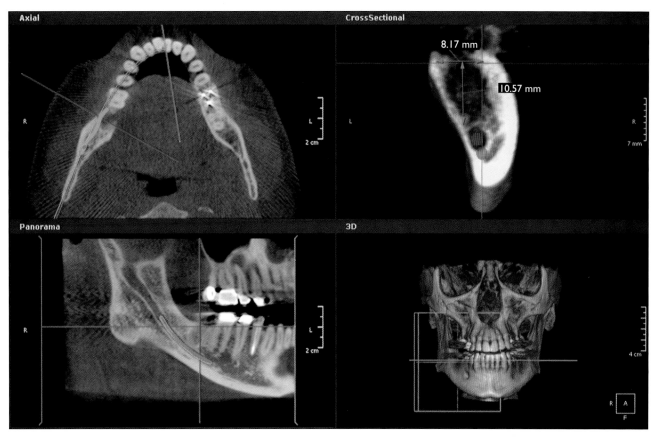

Fig 7-4c Here, the cortex of the bone is easily visualized using the Dental function and 3-D tools. The shape of the submandibular fossa is also apparent.

89

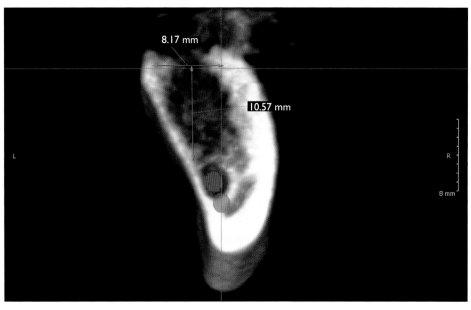

Fig 7-4d Close-up of the 7.5-mm cross section from Fig 7-4c. The two *red dots* demonstrate the change in position of the nerve canal from the posterior end of the slice *(upper dot)* to the anterior end of the slice *(lower dot)*.

REFERENCES

1. Danforth RA, Miles DA. Cone beam volume imaging (CBVI): 3D applications for dentistry. Ir Dent 2007;10(9):14–18.

2. Miles DA, Shelley RK. Pre-surgical implant site assessment: Part I–Precise and practical radiographic stent construction for cone beam CT imaging. LearnDigital website. Available at: http://www.learndigital.net/articles/2006/presurgical_stent.pdf. Accessed 14 July 2008.

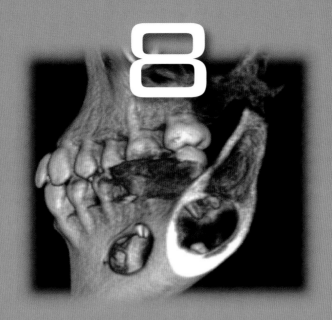

ODONTOGENIC LESIONS

Although many odontogenic cysts and tumors are rare, the application of cone beam volumetric imaging (CBVI) to characterize these lesions is invaluable for preoperative planning and clinical management.

FIG

8-1

SUPERNUMERARY TOOTH

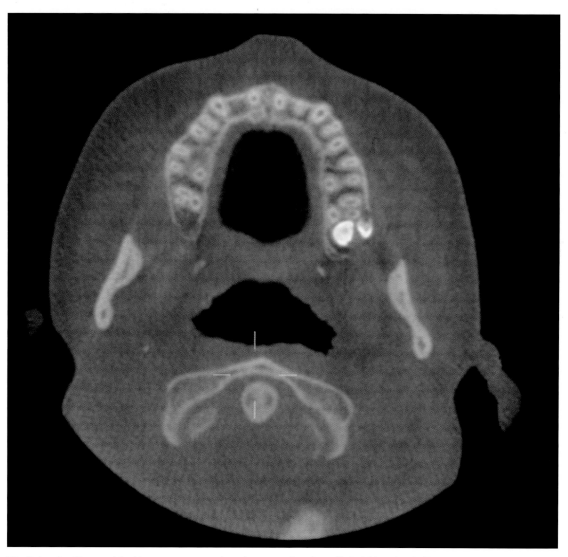

Fig 8-1a An 18-year-old white woman was referred to an oral and maxillofacial imaging facility in Seattle, Washington, for CBVI evaluation with respect to a suspected supernumerary tooth. The maxillary third molars had not yet erupted. The axial section shows the maxillary left third molar and associated supernumerary.

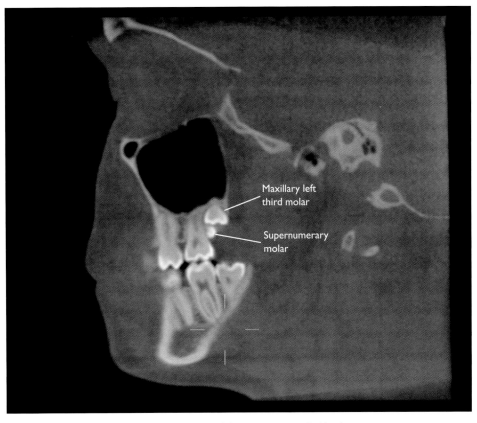

Fig 8-1b The sagittal section shows these teeth in a more recognizable view.

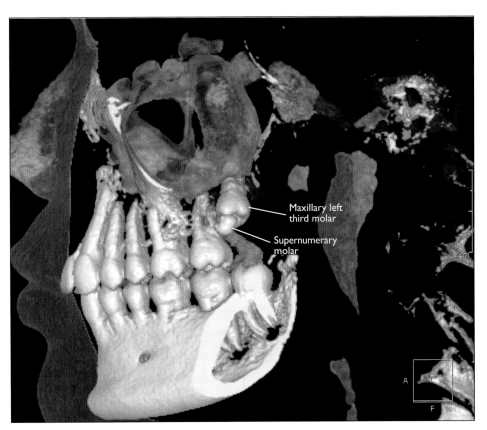

Fig 8-1c A 3-D grayscale reconstruction shows the orientation of the maxillary left third molar and supernumerary.

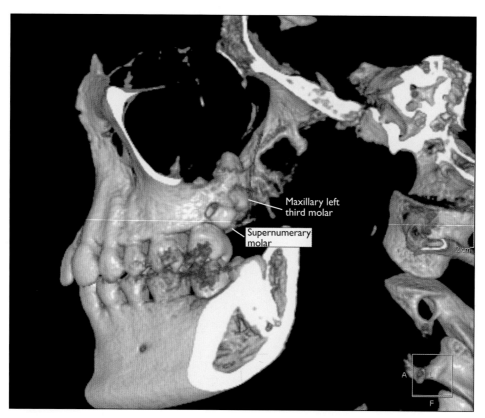

Fig 8-1d A 3-D color reconstruction shows the orientation of the tooth and supernumerary in relation to the bone.

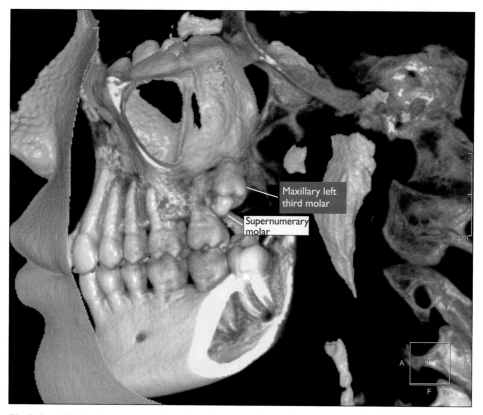

Fig 8-1e A 3-D color reconstruction shows the orientation of the tooth and supernumerary in relation to soft tissue structures such as the maxillary sinus and partial airway.

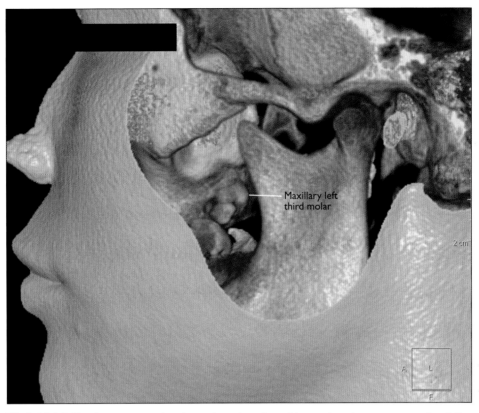

Fig 8-1f A 3-D color reconstruction shows the orientation of the tooth and supernumerary in relation to anatomic structures and facial soft tissues. The black box over the eyes is necessary to preserve the anonymity of the patient, since the facial detail is so remarkable.

95

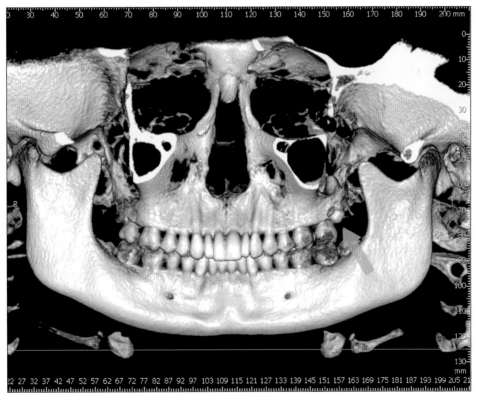

Fig 8-1g In this 3-D color panoramic reconstruction of the patient, note how single midline anatomic structures such as the hyoid bone and spine are still projected twice because of the image reconstruction process. The maxillary left third molar is marked *(arrow)*.

FIG
8-2

SIMPLE BONE CYST

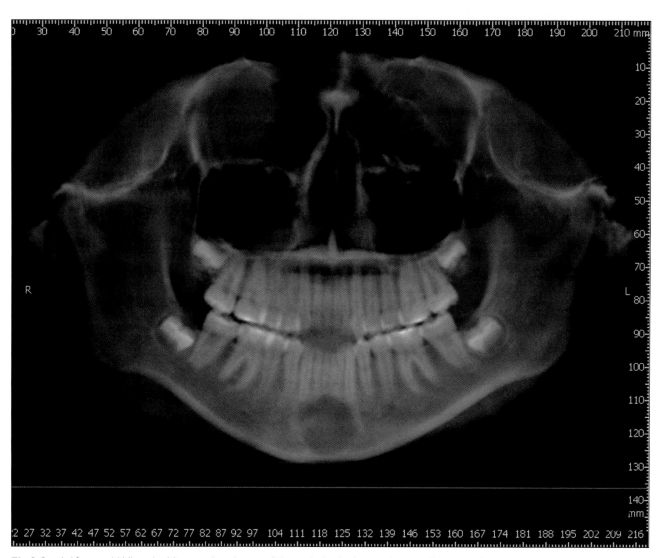

Fig 8-2a A 10-year-old Hispanic girl presenting a large radiolucent lesion in the anterior mandible was referred to the oral and maxillofacial imaging facility in the orthodontic department at the University of California, San Francisco, for CBVI evaluation. A panoramic-like image reconstructed from the cone beam data volume reveals a large, well-defined, circular radiolucency with a cortical border. No internal calcification or root resorption is apparent. There appears to be some remodeling of the inferior cortex of the mandible.

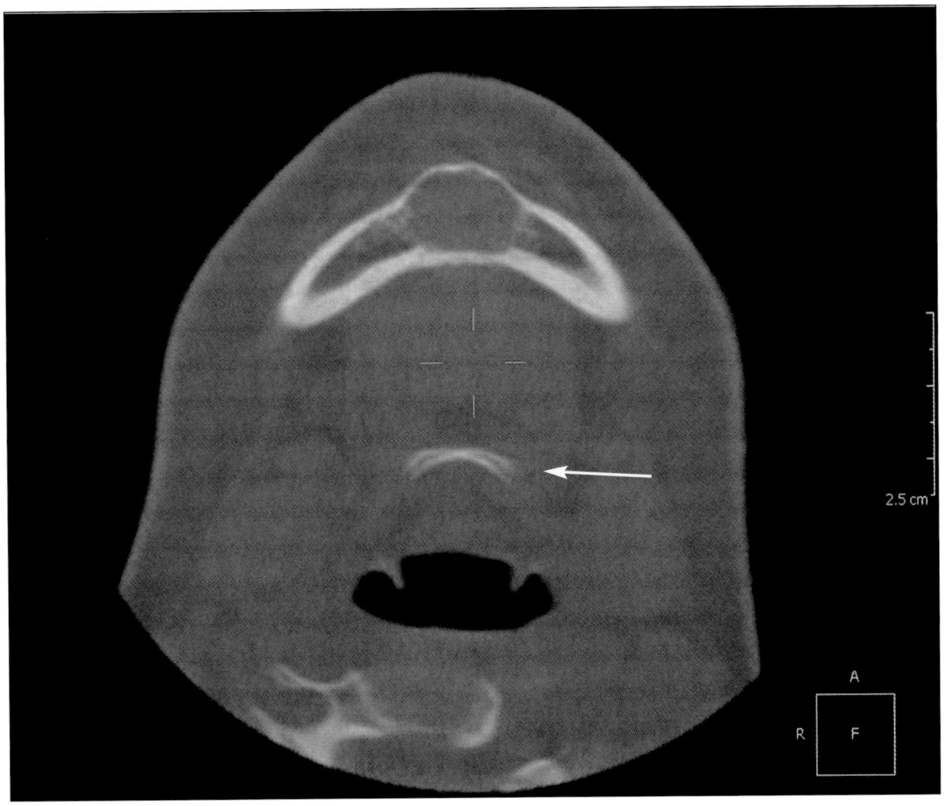

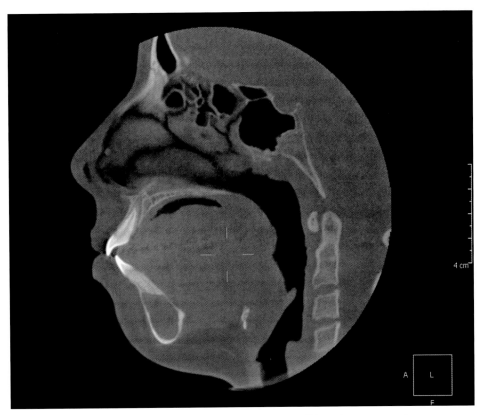

Fig 8-2b A thin axial slice at the level of the hyoid bone *(arrow)* reveals the expansile nature of the lesion *not* seen in the previous panoramic image.

Fig 8-2c A thin sagittal slice shows thinning of the anterior mandible and some expansion.

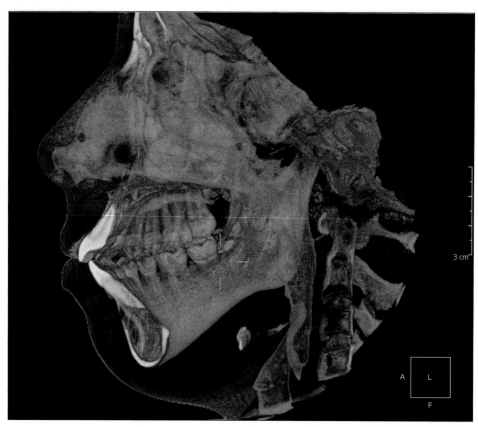

Fig 8-2d A sagittal slice (60.0 mm thick) rendered in 3-D color shows the lesion and soft tissue outlines. Note also the transparent airway and paranasal sinus regions.

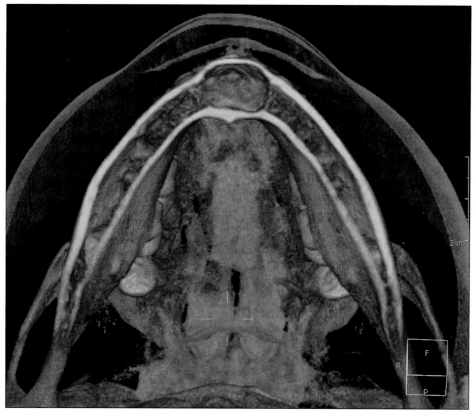

Fig 8-2e An axial slice (60.0 mm thick) rendered in 3-D color showing lesion and soft tissue outlines. Note also the transparent airway and paranasal sinus regions.

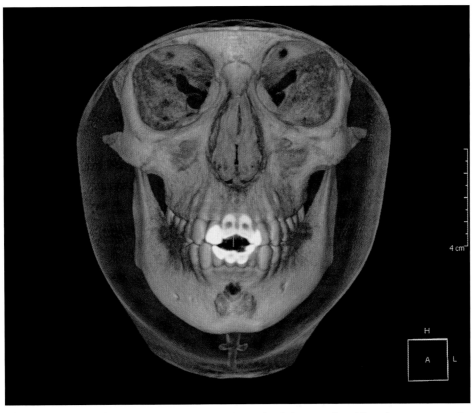

Fig 8-2f A full 3-D color rendering shows the lesion and soft tissue outlines. Note the apparent perforation of the anterior cortical bone. This is a pseudoperforation caused by the slice thickness. The cortex, though thinned, is intact, as seen in the previous images.

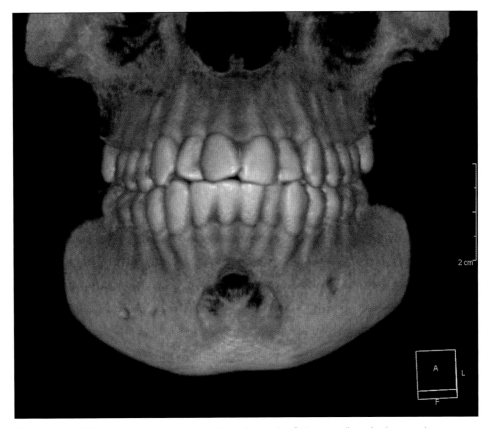

Fig 8-2g A full 3-D color rendering shows the lesion and soft tissue outlines. Again, note the apparent perforation of cortical bone. This image is fully rendered, so the "perforation" actually comes from the image processing. The opacity and transparency functions may have been manipulated incorrectly. All 2-D and 3-D image data must be examined to make a correct assessment.

FIG

8-3

NASOPALATINE DUCT CYST

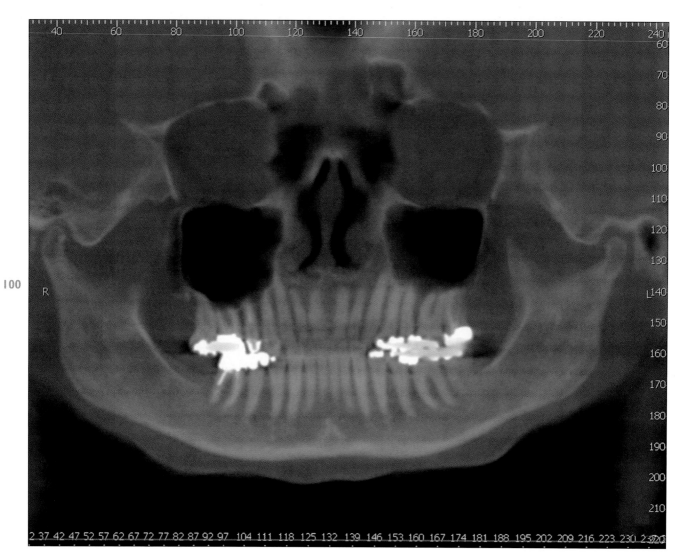

Fig 8-3a A 58-year-old white woman was referred for implant site assessment for replacement of the right mandibular second molar. The panoramic radiograph was not provided, but a typical reconstruction simulates what it would have shown; the reconstructed "panoramic" image fails to reveal the existence of the nasopalatine duct cyst in the anterior maxilla. This is a good example of the kind of occult pathology found in CBVI data volumes by oral and maxillofacial radiologists.

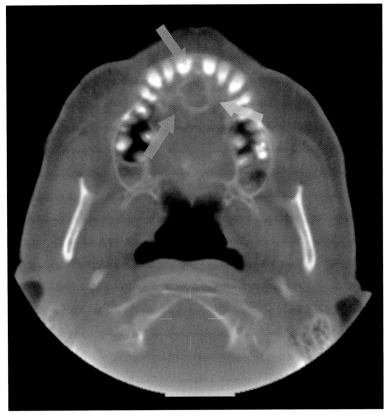

Fig 8-3b An axial image shows the size and irregular margins of the palatal cyst (*arrows*), indicating expansion.

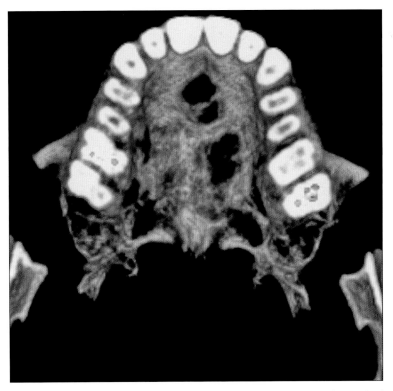

Fig 8-3c A 3-D color reconstruction suggests possible perforation of the palatal cyst. Recall that, as shown in Fig 8-2g, this apparent bone loss may be only an effect of the image processing.

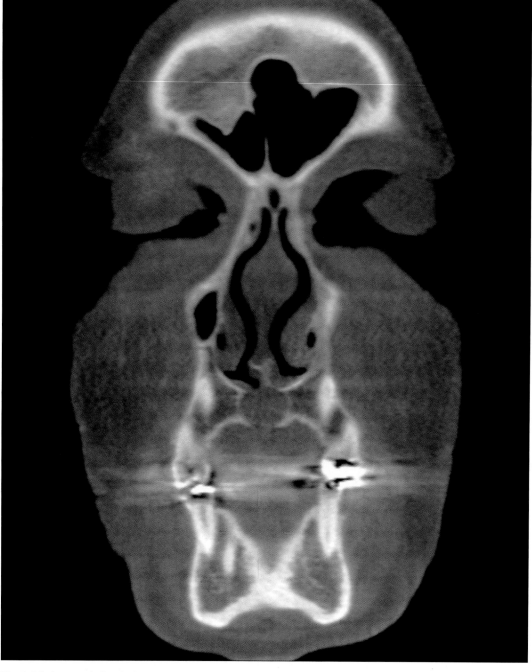

Fig 8-3d A coronal slice demonstrates the expansile nature of the lesion. Note that the lesion has already eroded the floor of the nasal fossa bilaterally.

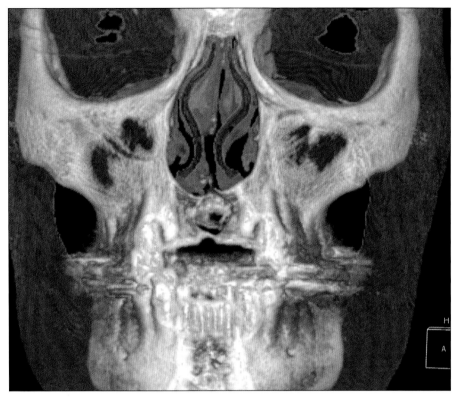

Fig 8-3e A coronal 3-D color rendering further suggests perforation of the buccal and possibly the palatal bones by the lesion.

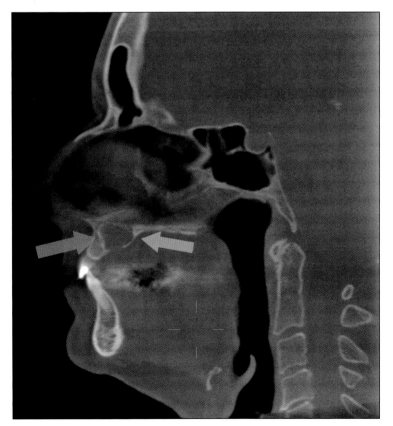

Fig 8-3f A sagittal slice demonstrates expansion and possible erosion of the inferior region of the palate, since the opening from the foramen *(arrows)* appears larger than normal.

104

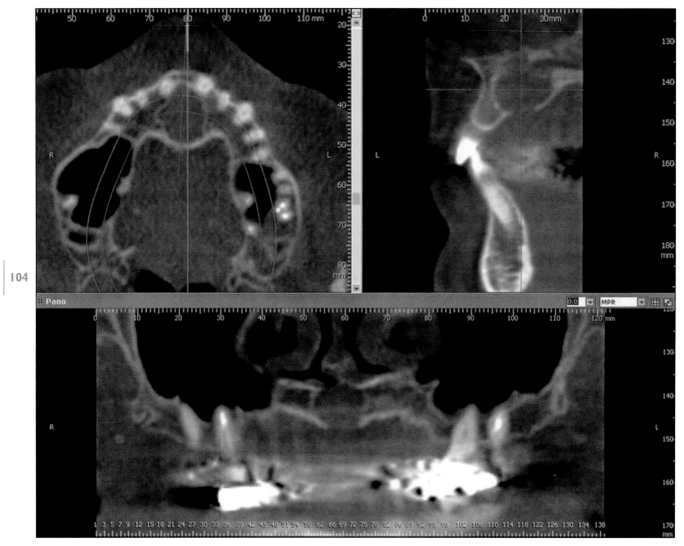

Fig 8-3g The Implant mode can be used to examine the central area of the lesion in all three planes of section.

FIG

8-4

ODONTOGENIC KERATOCYST

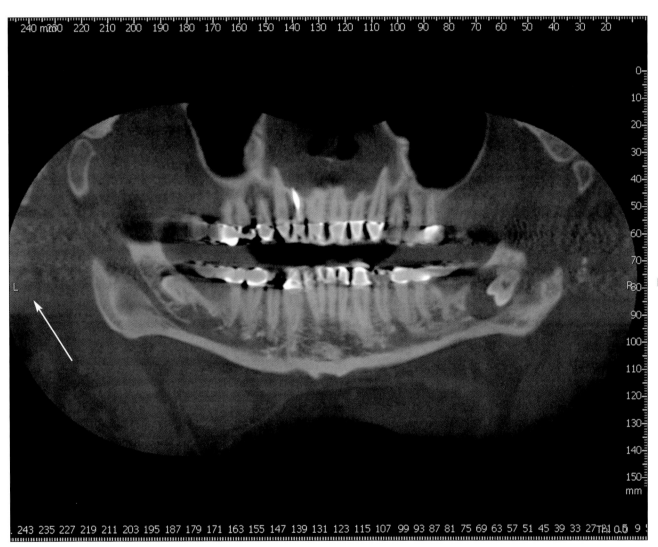

Fig 8-4a A 53-year-old white man was referred to Case Western Reserve University School of Dental Medicine in Cleveland, Ohio, for evaluation of an impacted third molar. No information was provided to the radiologist other than a request to study the data volume. There was no referral comment on the prescription form about a suspected cyst. This is a pseudopanoramic reconstruction slice (0.15 mm). At the time of this evaluation, the Preferences section of the software had been programmed to display the image in a reverse format; that is, with the patient's left side *on the left (white arrow)*. The lesion actually surrounds the mandibular right third molar.

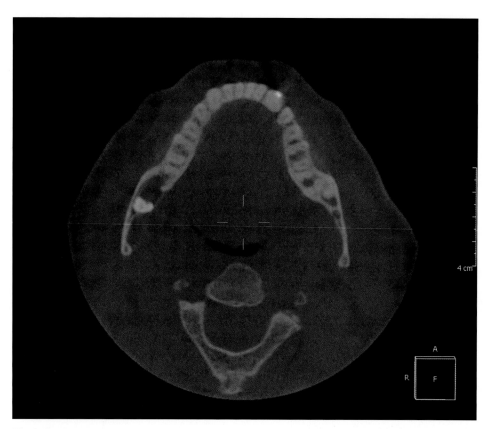

Fig 8-4b An axial view shows the pericoronal nature and expansion of the lesion, resulting in remodeling of the lingual cortex.

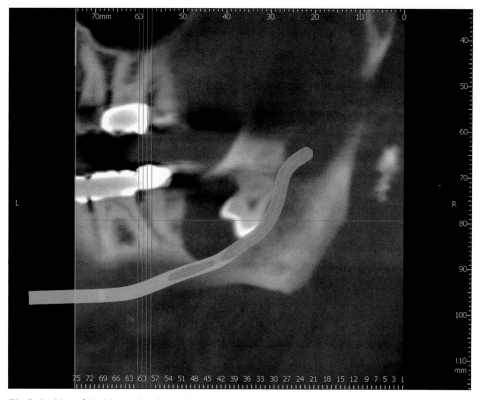

Fig 8-4c Use of the Nerve drawing tool in the Implant mode to determine the relationship of the tooth and lesion to the inferior alveolar canal. *Orange* represents the nerve outside the plane of section. *Green* represents the nerve in the particular plane of section.

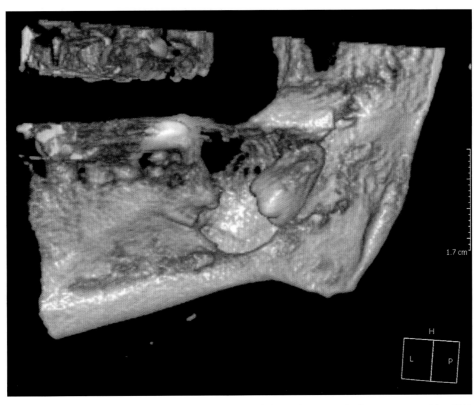

Fig 8-4d By selecting the Cube tool in the software, this image is automatically reconstructed in a 3-D color rendering. The clinician or operator can also change the coloration by selecting Presets, which can be created and stored in the program by assigning different colors and opacity and transparency values to particular voxels.

107

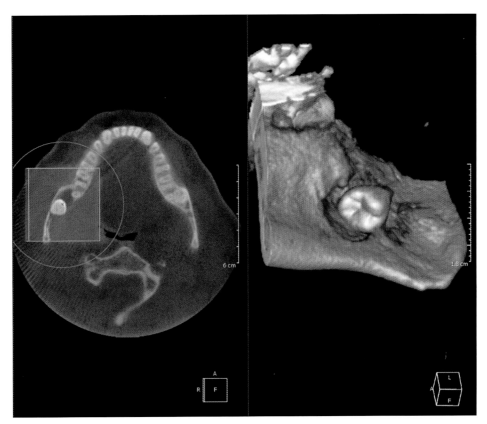

Fig 8-4e By selecting the Cube tool, the image can be rotated in 3-D to demonstrate the occlusal surface anatomy.

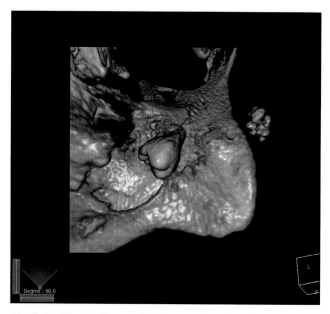

Fig 8-4f A similar, but isolated, view of the image from Fig 8-4e has been rotated to view the inferior extent of the lesion in 3-D color. Note the linear resorptive pattern of the right mandibular second molar here and in Fig 8-4e.

Fig 8-4g The OnDemand 3D server-based platform software (CyberMed International) also has an Endoscope tool that allows the visualization of even more detail of this lesion. The cauliflower-like radiopaque object posterior to the ramus is a calcified lymph node.

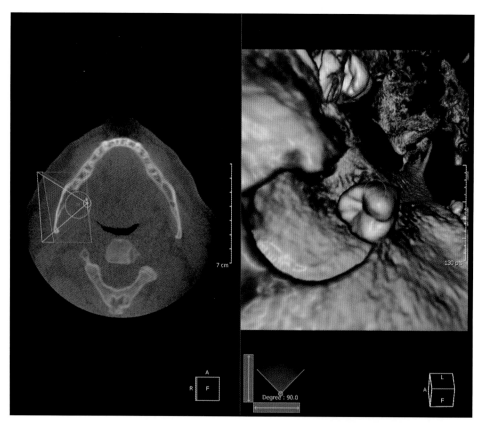

Fig 8-4h Applying the Endoscope tool and rotating the image displays the occlusal surface even more precisely.

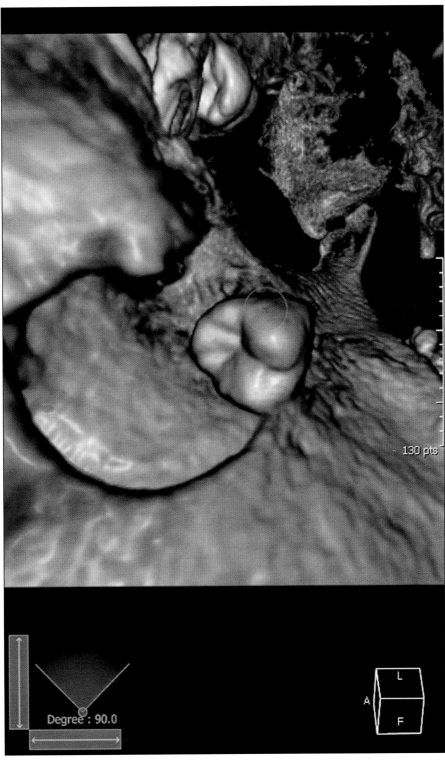

Fig 8-4i An enlarged, isolated image captured from the right side of Fig 8-4h. This is done within the program with a Capture tool. All images captured can be stored as compressed JPEG, TIFF, or bitmap images. The size of a compressed JPEG image is often less than 400 kB. Note that there is no loss of image quality, even in this enlarged view.

FIG
8-5

PERICORONAL RADIOLUCENCY

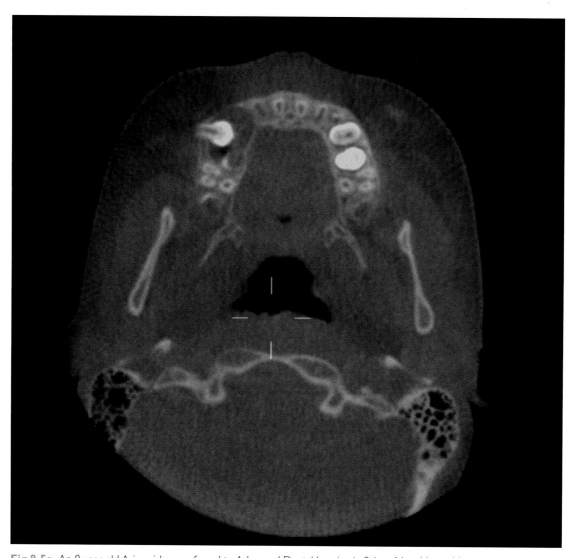

Fig 8-5a An 8-year-old Asian girl was referred to Advanced Dental Imaging in Salem, New Hampshire, to evaluate a radiolucency in the right anterior maxilla. The axial view through the midroot section of the maxillary dentition reveals a large, expansile, well-defined pericoronal radiolucency around the maxillary right canine, which was impacted and displaced superiorly against the lateral wall of the right nasal fossa. The radiolucency has a definitive cortical border.

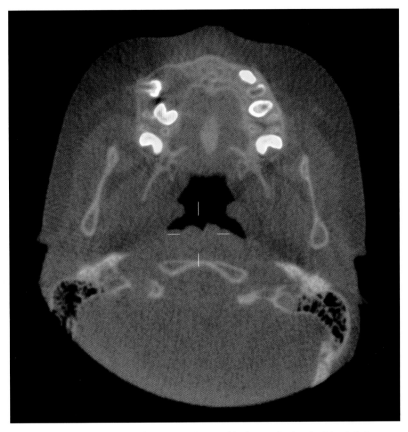

Fig 8-5b Another axial view of the pericoronal lesion at the level of the inferior portion of the condylar heads.

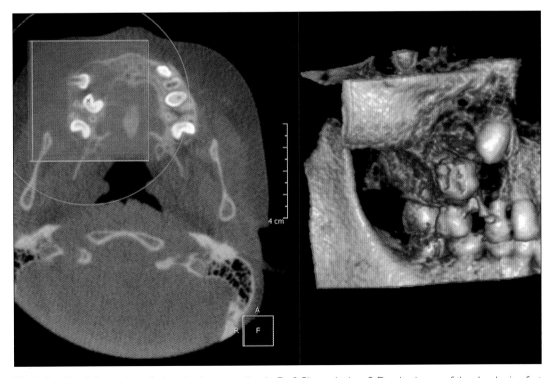

Fig 8-5c The Cube tool applied to the image section in Fig 8-5b results in a 3-D color image of the developing first premolar in its deviated orientation. The view is of the developing root structure from the facial side. The lesion has displaced the first and second permanent premolars. The maxillary right first premolar had completed only about one-third of its root formation. A linear resorption pattern is seen on the roots of the primary canine and primary first molar.

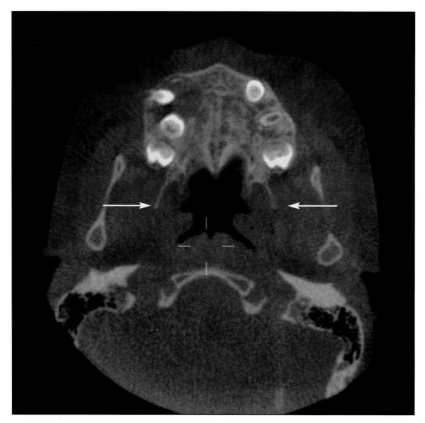

Fig 8-5d A more superior slice at the level of the lateral pterygoid plates *(white arrows)*.

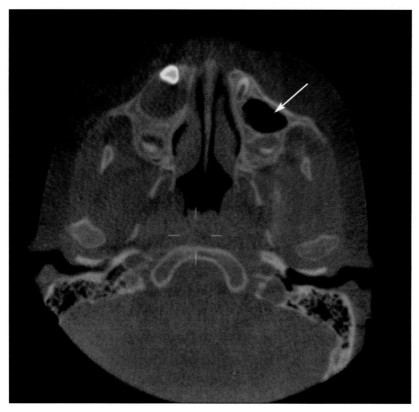

Fig 8-5e An axial slice shows the lesion at the level of the developing permanent canine crown. The lesion obviously extends to the maxillary sinus region. The *white arrow* indicates the left antrum.

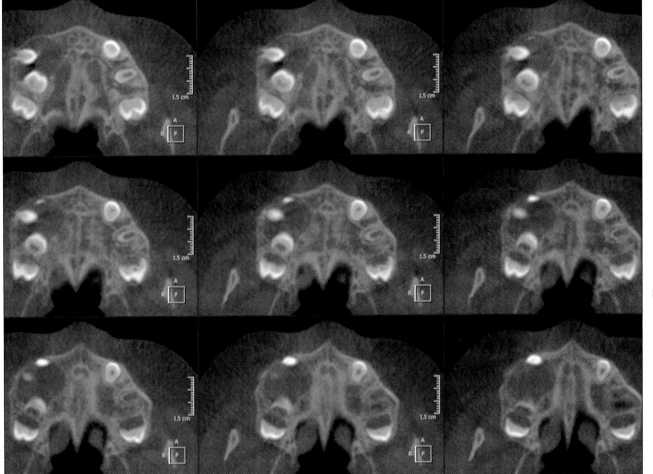

Fig 8-5f A typical 9 × 9 series, like traditional computerized tomography, shows the axial views at 1.0-mm slices from the level of the developing premolar crowns to the incisal tip of the maxillary right canine.

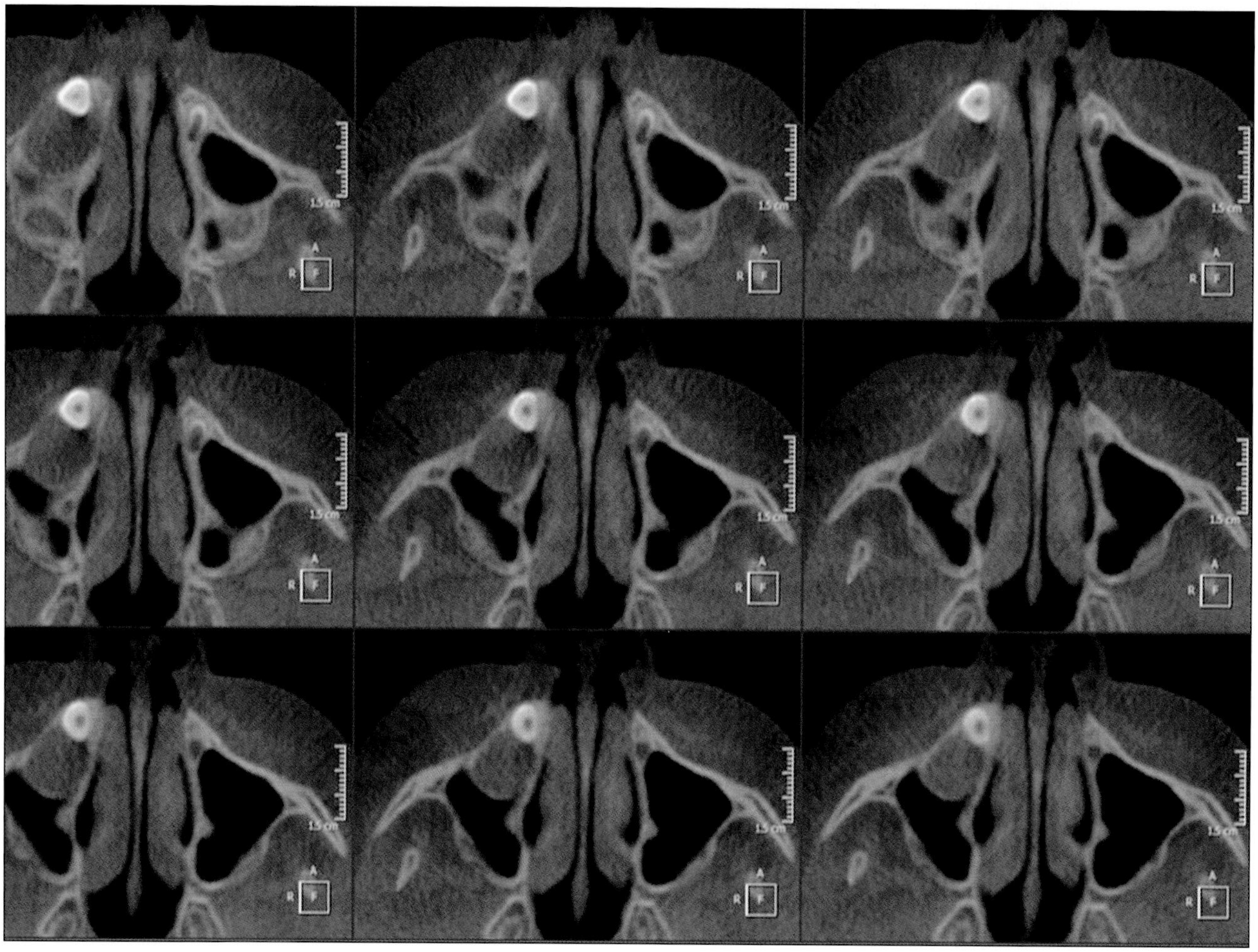

Fig 8-5g Another 9 × 9 series, continuing the axial views at 1.0-mm slice thickness, shows extension into the maxillary sinus and the relationship of the maxillary right canine to the root structure. Note the distinct cortical margin.

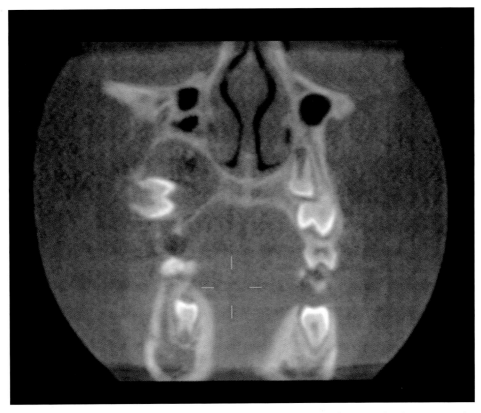

Fig 8-5h A coronal section through the midcrown region of the ectopic first premolar demonstrates the buccal expansion of the lesion. There are no apparent internal calcifications, even at this slice thickness of 1.0 mm.

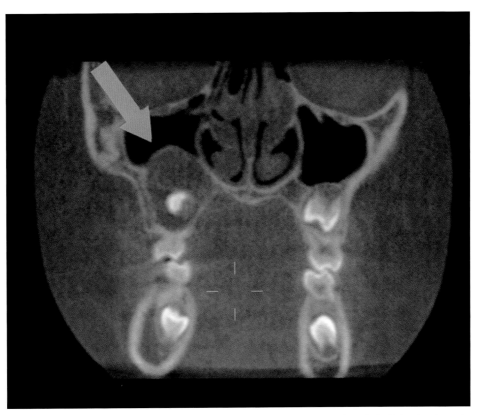

Fig 8-5i A more posterior coronal section shows the cortical definition of the lesion's border *(arrow)*.

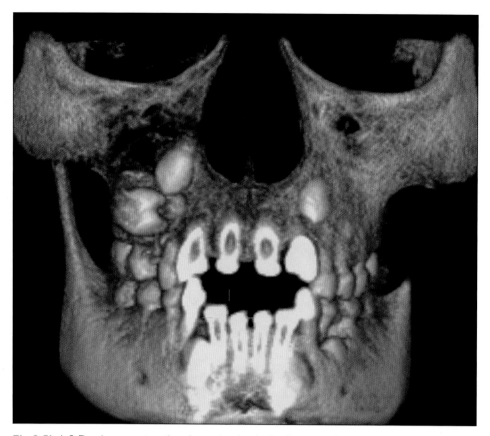

Fig 8-5j A 3-D color reconstruction shows the developing first premolar crown in precise relation to the incisal tip of the developing maxillary right canine. The lesion extends from the right lateral incisor region through the maxilla and into the maxillary right sinus midway up the nose. Posteriorly, it reaches the first molar region.

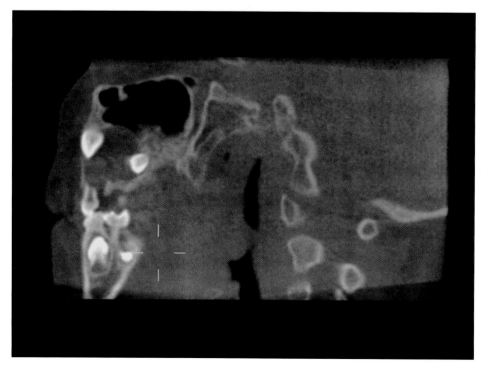

Fig 8-5k A sagittal view shows the displacement of the canine and premolar as well as extension into the maxillary sinus region.

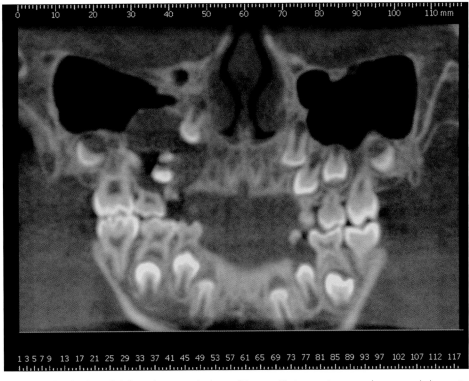

Fig 8-5l The Arch tool defines the central plane of the maxilla to create a pseudopanoramic image to visualize the internal contents of the lesion.

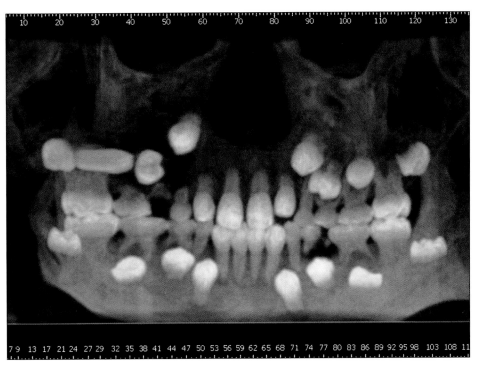

Fig 8-5m This maximum intensity projection image demonstrates the difficulty in orienting the structures correctly from a panoramic-type view.

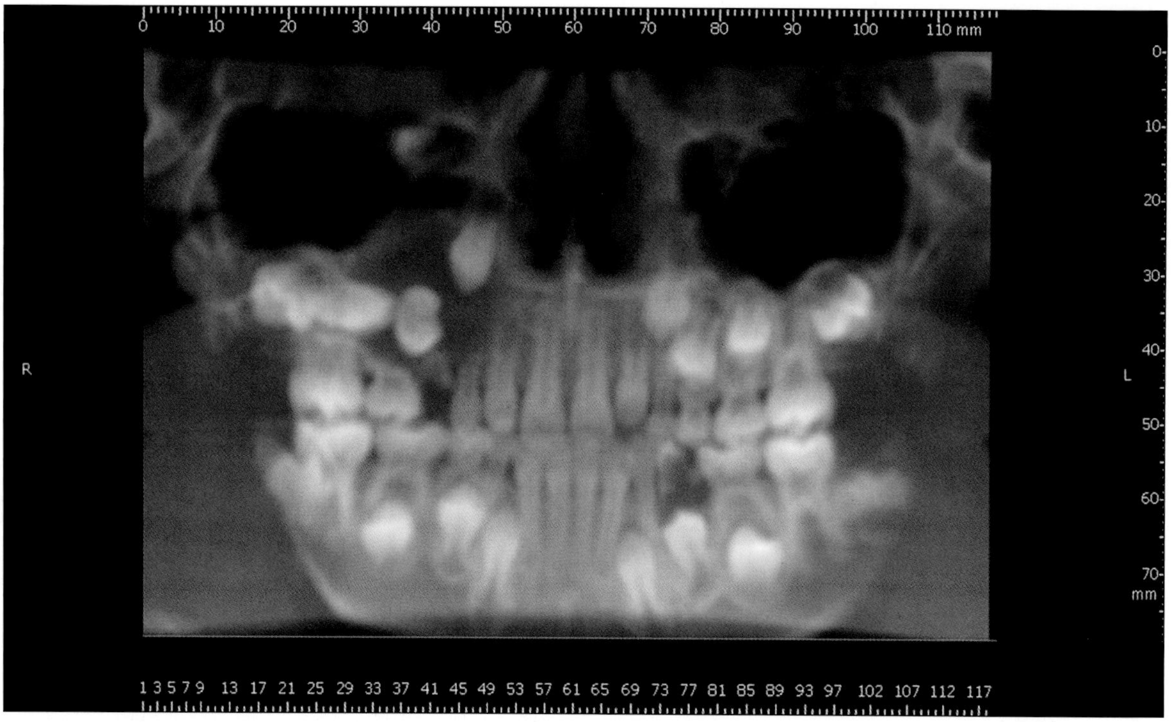

Fig 8-5n A reconstructed panoramic image at a thickness of 20.0 mm. Note that this type of image would be deficient for any clinician to fully characterize the lesion. The cortical margin is not appreciated, and the precise orientation of the first premolar is not discernible.

Differential diagnosis, Fig 8-5

Although the lesion contained no discernible internal calcifications, the most likely odontogenic lesion would be an adenomatoid odontogenic tumor. The sex of the patient, location of the lesion, resorptive pattern, and tooth displacement suggest this type of lesion. Additional possible diagnoses would include an odontogenic keratocyst and an ameloblastic fibroma. Since an ameloblastic fibroma behaves like a fibroma and rarely recurs, it can be treated much more conservatively than an ameloblastoma. Incisional biopsy prior to surgical removal was indicated to determine the precise histology of the lesion for preoperative planning.

Fig

8-6

MANDIBULAR RADIOLUCENCY

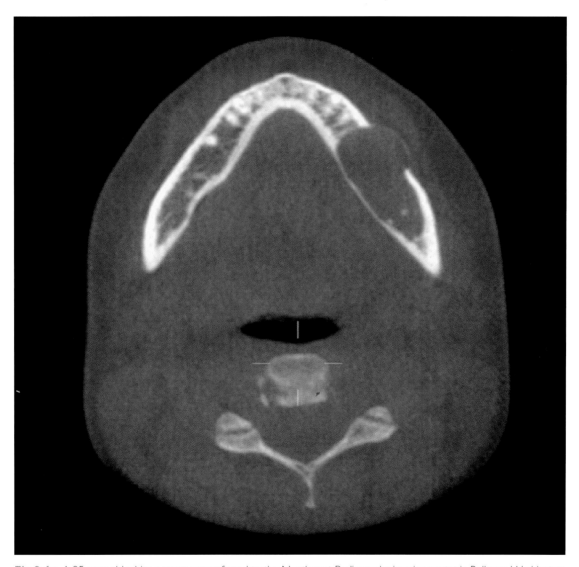

Fig 8-6a A 25-year-old white woman was referred to the Northwest Radiography imaging center in Bellevue, Washington, for evaluation of a lesion in the left posterior mandible. An axial slice shows a large, solitary, well-defined expansile lesion with a cortical outline in the inferior portion of the left mandible. There is no apparent perforation, but the cortex is significantly thinned in this slice. One or two opacities are seen within the lesion.

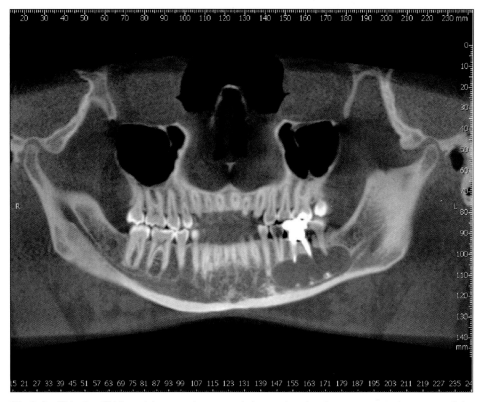

Fig 8-6b This coronal section confirms both the expansion of the lesion and the thinning of the lingual cortex *(arrow)*. The lesion is close to the molar roots of the mandibular left first molar, which had previously undergone root canal therapy.

Fig 8-6c This slice (0.15 mm) is a pseudopanoramic image showing the anteroposterior extent of the lesion from the mandibular left canine to the region of the third molar. The cortical border undulates around the second premolar, first molar, and second molar. Note the small diffuse radiopacities within the lesion at its inferior margin, as well as as the displacement of the inferior alveolar nerve.

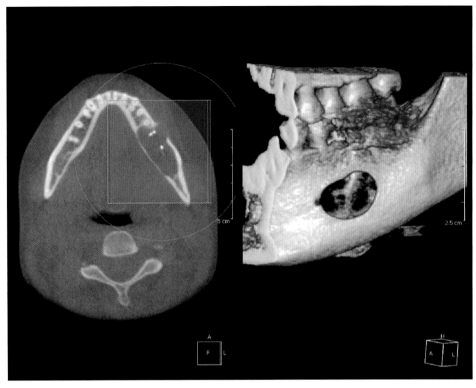

Fig 8-6d The Cube tool was used to visualize the perforation of the buccal cortex by the lesion in a 3-D color view.

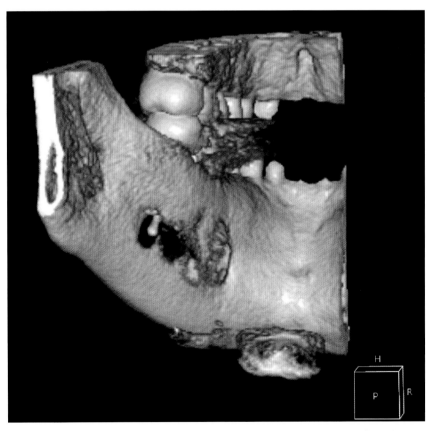

Fig 8-6e The lingual cortex in this patient also appears to be perforated. The small opacity seen at the apex of the first molar represents some endodontic fill material.

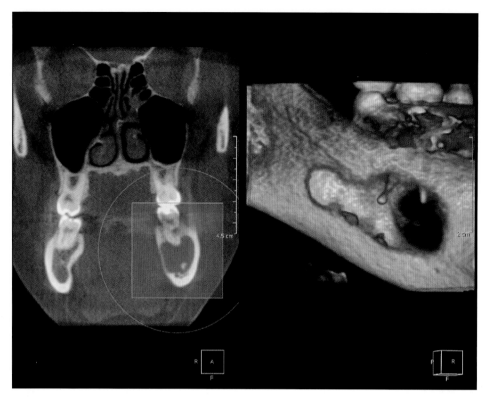

Fig 8-6f The Cube tool is used to create a 3-D color image of the lingual area and internal region of the lesion.

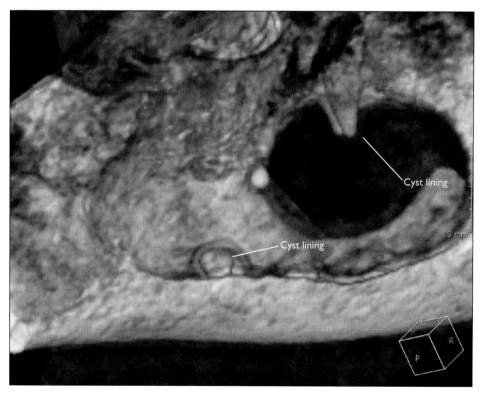

Fig 8-6g In this software, the clinician or radiologist can apply Presets (combinations of colors, opacities, and transparencies) to the histogram region of selected tissues. In this patient, these Presets have revealed a thin soft tissue layer similar to a cyst lining around the molar apex and over the bony enostosis at the inferior cortical margin.

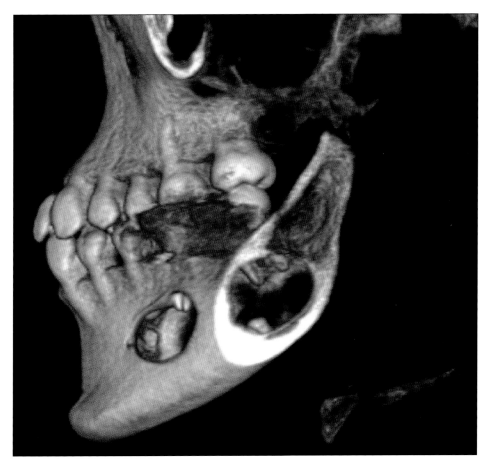

Fig 8-6h A 3-D color reconstruction of the same lesion from the lateral view.

124

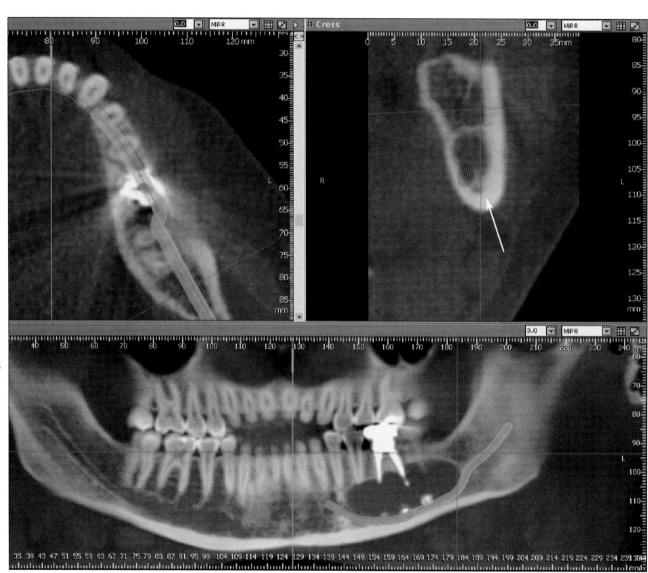

Fig 8-6i The Arch and Nerve tools are used *(top left)* to define the central plane of the mandible and locate the inferior alveolar nerve *(green line)*, as well as *(top right)* to create a cross-sectional image of the lesion. The reference line *(white arrow)* shows the cross-sectional slice where the inferior alveolar nerve *(red dot)* begins to dip below the lesion at its posterior border.

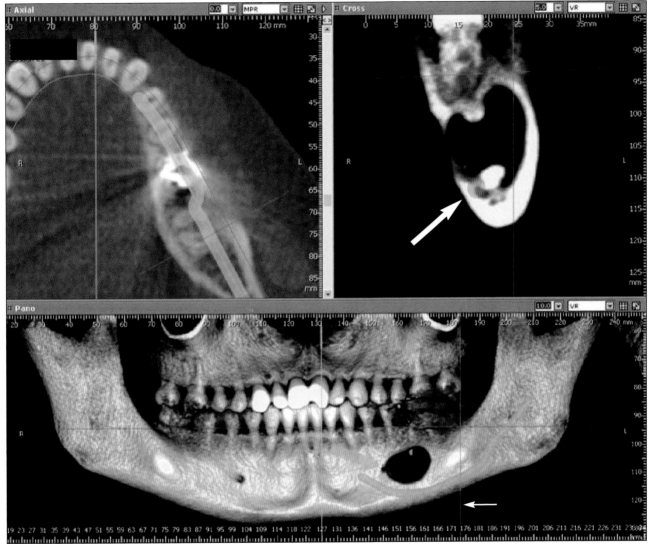

Fig 8-6j *(bottom panel)* The reference line *(small white arrow)* within the panoramic slice in a 3-D color reconstruction reveals where the inferior alveolar nerve *(orange line)* touches the area of enostosis. The *blue arrow* points to the perforation of the buccal cortex.

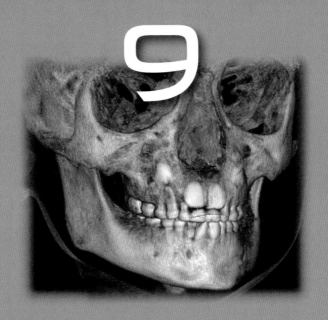

ORTHODONTIC ASSESSMENT

This section is *not* intended to present traditional orthodontic case workups; instead, it simply demonstrates a few cases where cone beam volumetric imaging (CBVI) information would help a clinician visualize the primary case problems. No analyses are presented or suggested.

FIG
9-1
ERUPTION OF MANDIBULAR PERMANENT TEETH

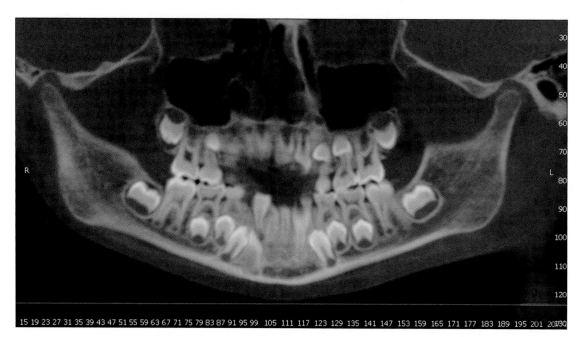

Fig 9-1a A 7-year-old boy was referred to an imaging service in Seattle, Washington, because of an unusual presentation of erupting mandibular permanent teeth. A reconstructed pseudopanoramic image shows a possible problem in the right anterior region of the mandible.

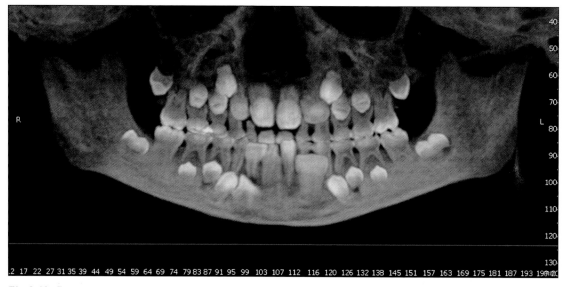

Fig 9-1b Even this maximum intensity projection (MIP) image does not accurately demonstrate the mandibular problem. A supernumerary right lateral incisor is suggested. The left lateral incisor appears to be "twinned" or possibly fused to another extra tooth.

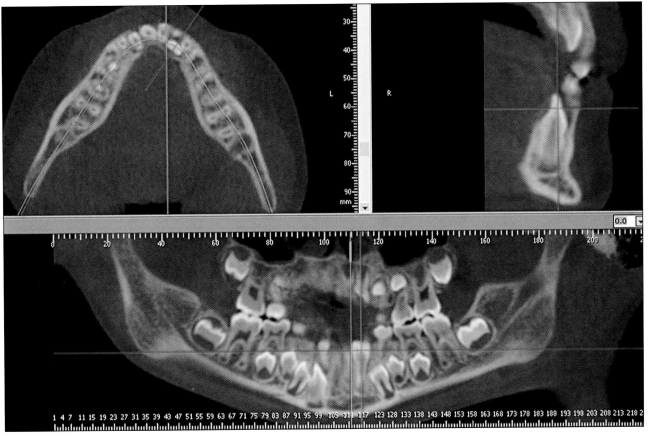

Fig 9-1c Instead of the fused tooth suggested in Fig 9-1b, the left lateral incisor is actually a normal tooth. Figure 9-1b had an arch curve selected that was too wide, which resulted in an inaccurate reconstruction. The axial and sagittal views show a normal lateral incisor.

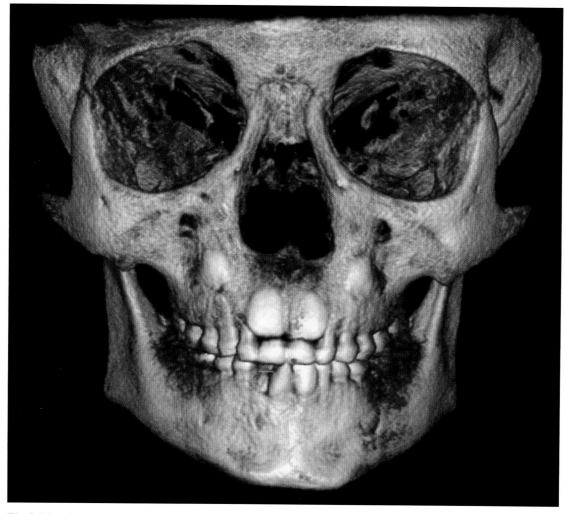

Fig 9-1d A 3-D color reconstruction showing the anterior region reveals that the mandibular right central incisor has erupted with an abnormal rotation.

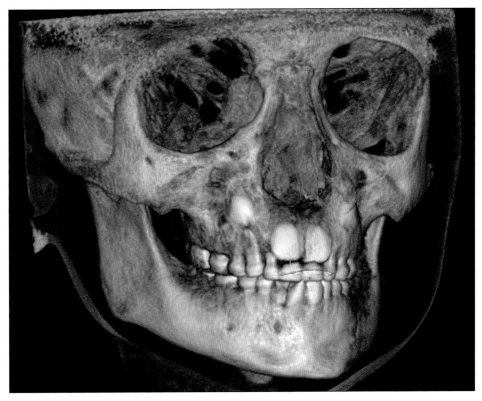

Fig 9-1e A 3-D color reconstruction in a profile configuration helps the clinician visualize the problem.

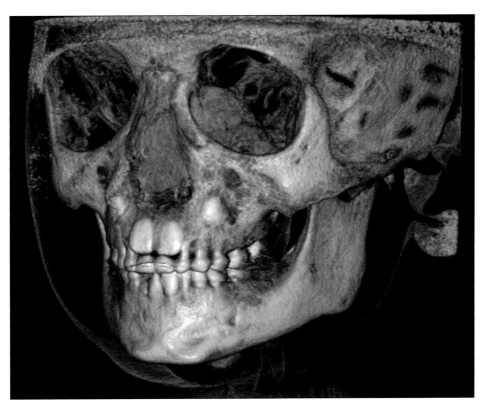

Fig 9-1f A 3-D color reconstruction in a profile configuration is created on the left side for comparison.

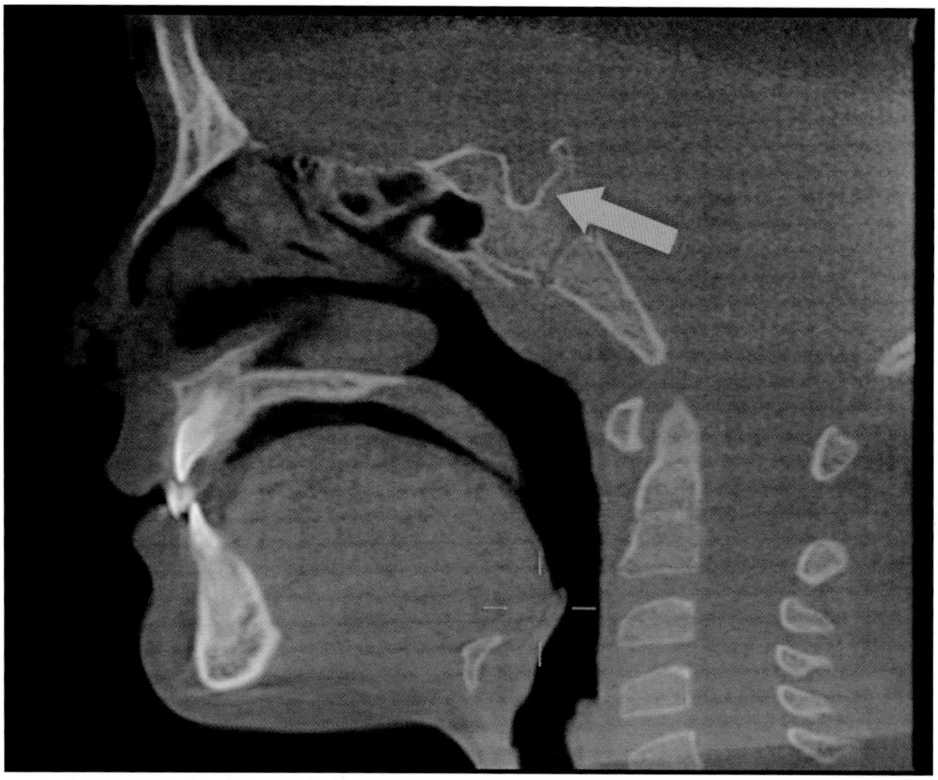

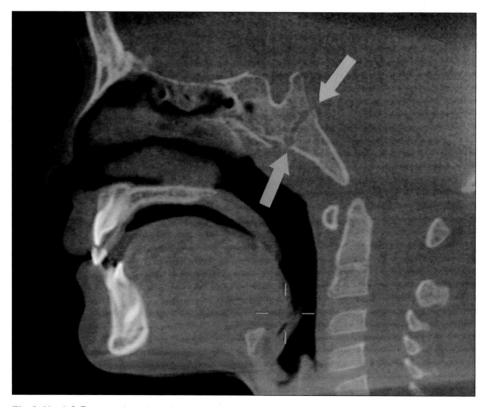

Fig 9-1g A 2-D grayscale sagittal view shows an unusual shape to the sella turcica *(blue arrow)*. The patient has no known endocrine or genetic abnormality. The finding, while reportable, is inconsequential in this case.

Fig 9-1h A 2-D grayscale sagittal view shows the development of the clivus *(blue arrows)*. This is a normal finding at this stage, but is never seen in the conventional panoramic views used by orthodontists.

FIG

9-2

PALATAL IMPACTION

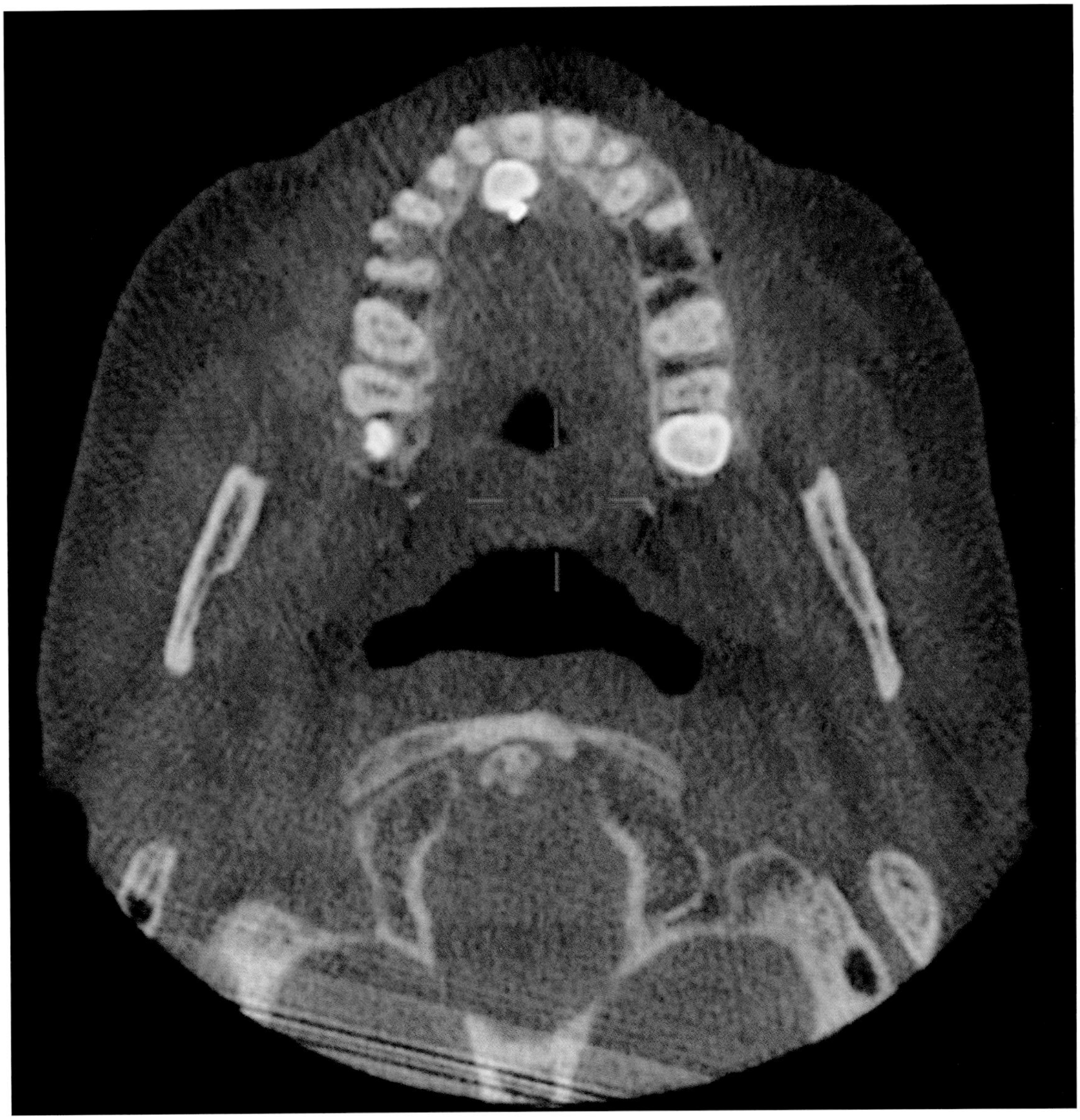

Fig 9-2a This is a case of a palatal impaction of a canine in a 23-year-old white man with retained primary molars. A temporary anchorage device had been employed to obtain traction in a previously unobtainable location. A 2-D grayscale axial view shows the palatally impacted maxillary right canine.

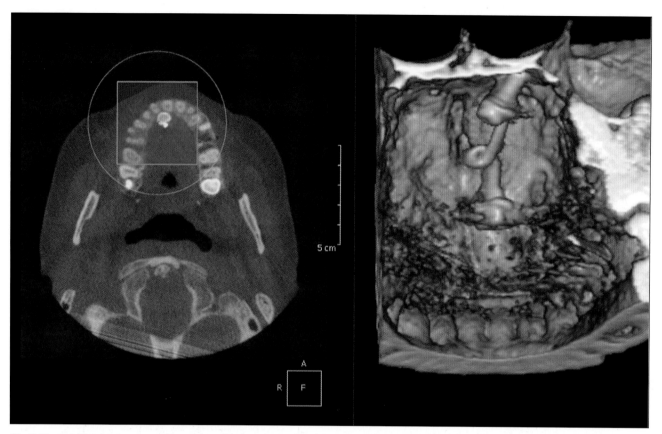

Fig 9-2b A 3-D color reconstruction of the axial view shows the anchorage device.

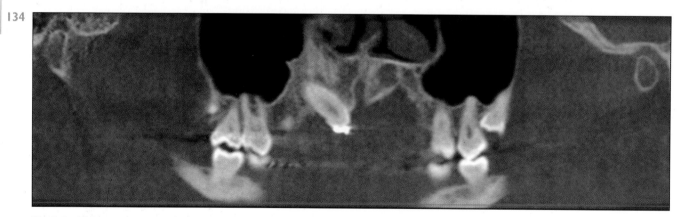

Fig 9-2c This pseudopanoramic reconstruction slice (0.15 mm) shows the canine, with its bracket, near the midline. Note the impacted maxillary left third molar in this plane.

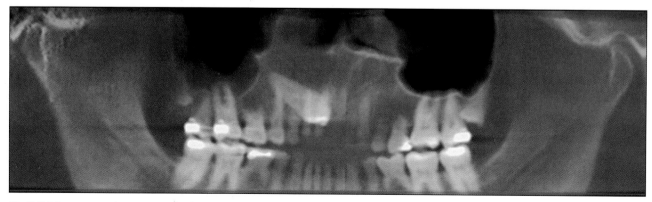

Fig 9-2d In a panoramic reconstruction including the impacted tooth, the actual bracket is barely visible.

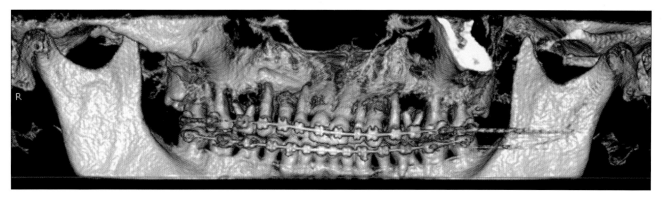

Fig 9-2e A 3-D color panoramic reconstruction shows the impacted canine and retained primary molars.

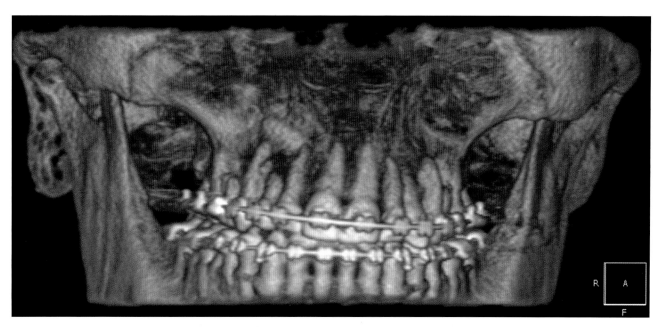

Fig 9-2f A 3-D color reconstruction reveals the position of the canine relative to the lateral incisor apex. Some transparency was used to show this relationship.

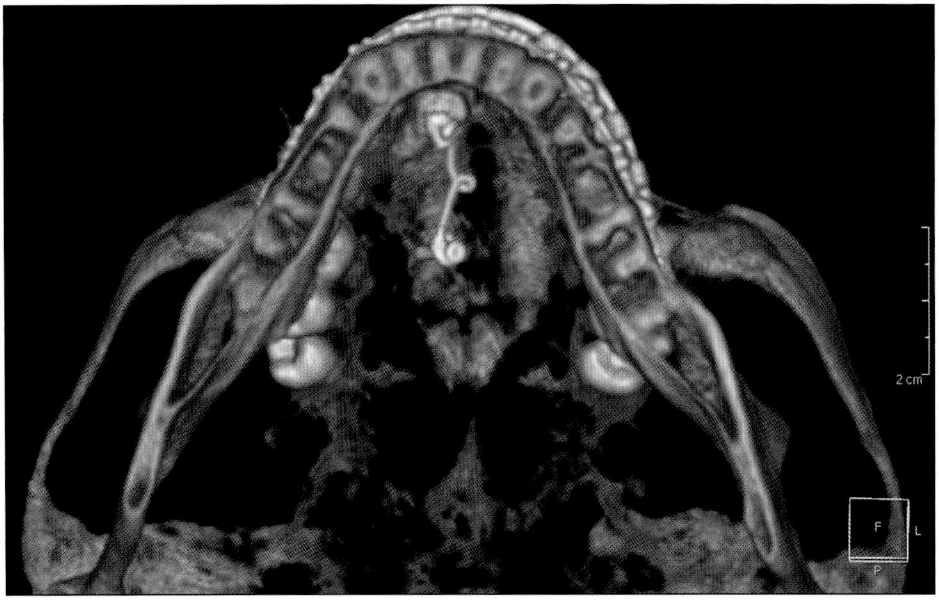

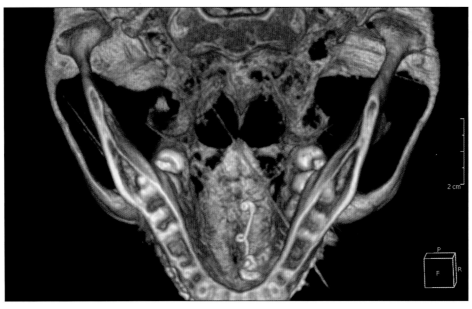

Fig 9-2g A slab 3-D color rendering (approximately 40 mm) in the axial plane uses transparency to show canine position.

Fig 9-2h A 3-D color reconstruction viewed from the foot end was created for the entire volume and shows the condyle/fossa relationships.

FIG

9-3

FACIAL ASYMMETRY

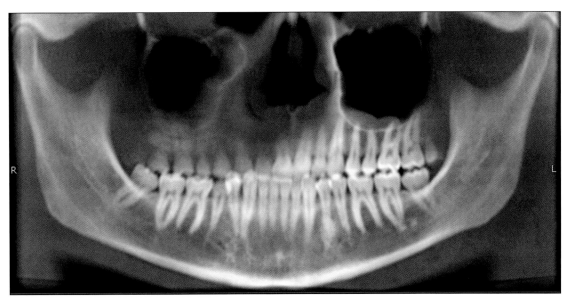

Fig 9-3a A 28-year-old white man was referred to the Northwest Radiography imaging center in Bellevue, Washington, for radiographic evaluation of his facial asymmetry and Class III malocclusion as part of his orthodontic records workup. In this panoramic image, the maxillary right teeth are not in the focal trough because of the patient's cross-bite. Note the shadow of thickened mucosa in the left antrum.

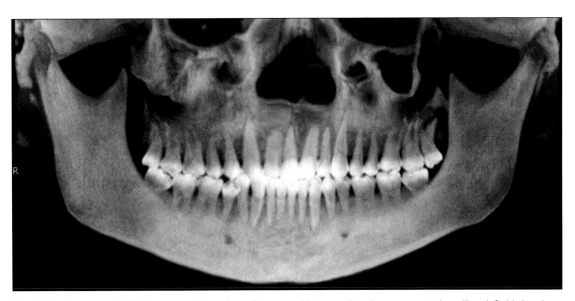

Fig 9-3b A panoramic MIP image provides a view of the cross-bite, as well as the overerupted maxillary left third molar.

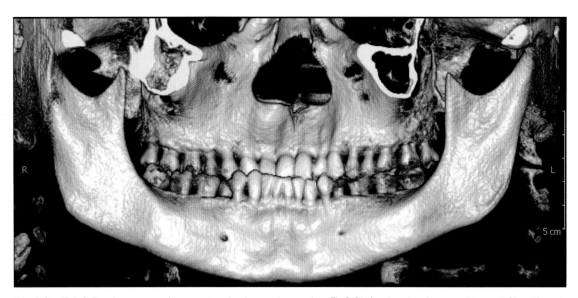

Fig 9-3c This 3-D color panoramic reconstruction is even better than Fig 9-3b for showing the cross-bite and Class III tooth relationships.

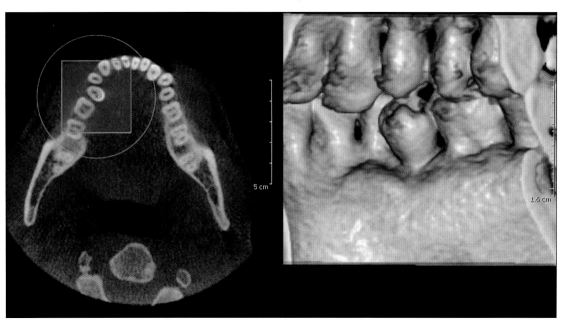

Fig 9-3d The Cube tool *(left)* renders a selected portion of the mandible to show the ectopic position of the mandibular right second premolar from the lingual aspect *(right)*.

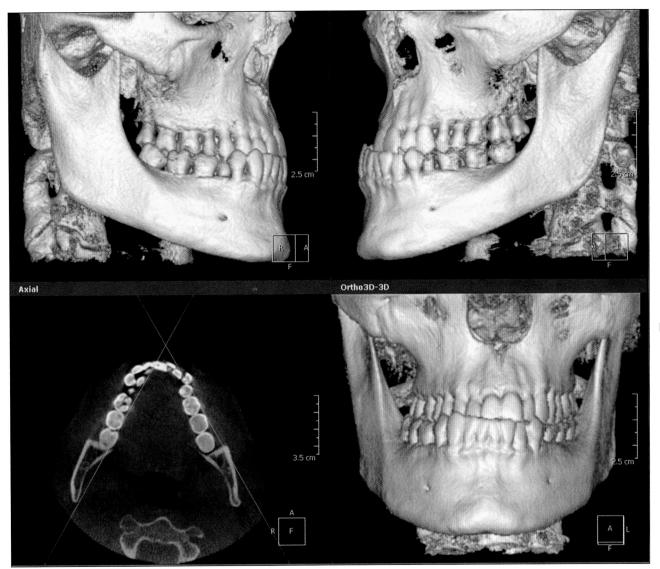

Fig 9-3e The Ortho Skeletal tool shows the tooth relationships from the lateral *(top left and right)* and facial *(bottom right)* views.

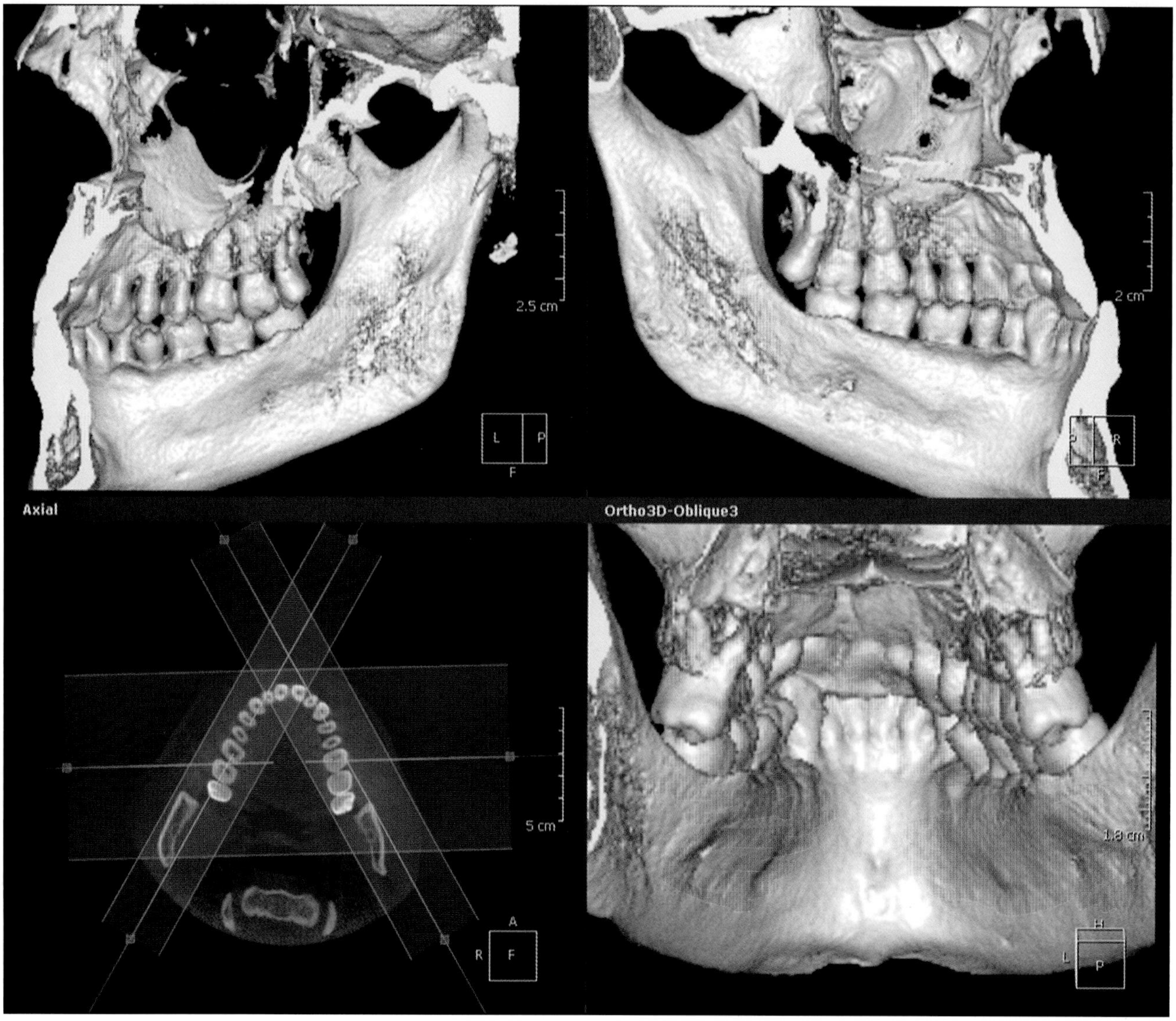

Fig 9-3f The 3-D Dentition tool uses the patient data to show the occlusion from the palatal surfaces.

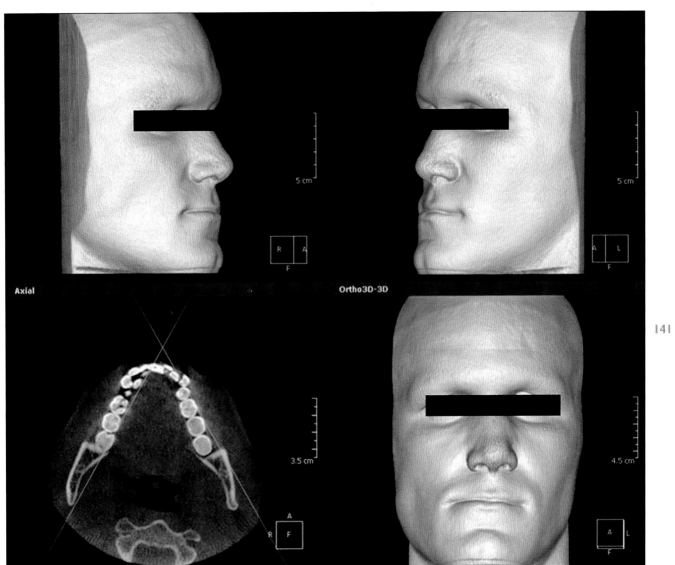

Fig 9-3g The 3-D Skin tool in the OnDemand 3D software (CyberMed International) shows the patient's asymmetric facial outline.

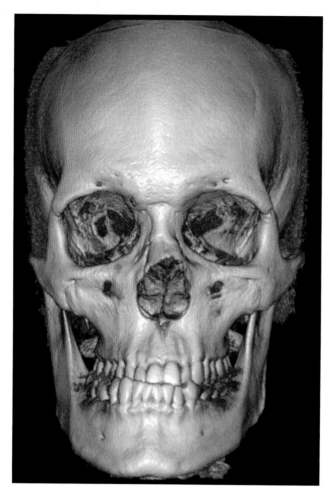

Fig 9-3h The cross-bite and midline deviation of the patient's mandible suggest right-side hyperplasia.

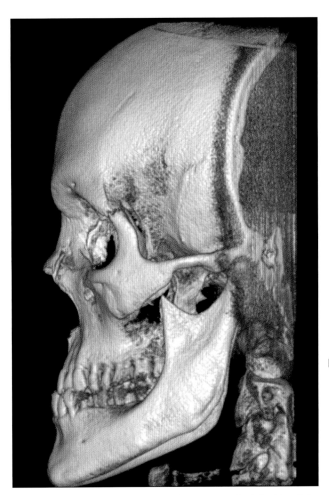

Figs 9-3i and 9-3j Comparison views confirm that the right side of the patient's mandible *(left)* is enlarged relative to the left side of the mandible *(right)*.

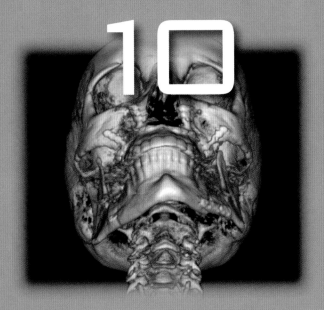

10

ORTHOGNATHIC SURGERY AND TRAUMA IMAGING

Since preoperative planning is best accomplished with accurate information about the morphology of the bony structures to be realigned, cone beam volumetric imaging (CBVI) is ideal for these cases. 2-D and 3-D grayscale and color information can accurately identify the anatomic architecture beneath a patient's soft tissue. Postoperatively, the screws, plates, implants, and the surgical outcomes can also be assessed. Even with the presence of scatter artifacts from the metallic materials often used, the images acquired from the data are remarkable.

FIG
10-1

FACIAL ASYMMETRY: PREOPERATIVE/ ORTHODONTIC EVALUATION

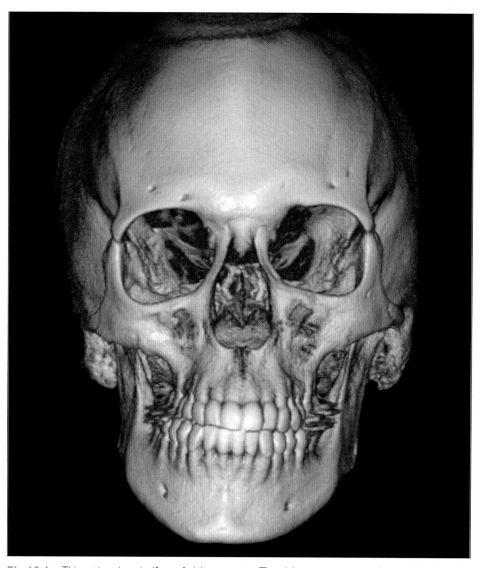

Fig 10-1a This patient has significant facial asymmetry. The right ramus appears shorter than the left. There is a right posterior cross-bite from the canine to the second molar and a significant midline deviation to the right side as well.

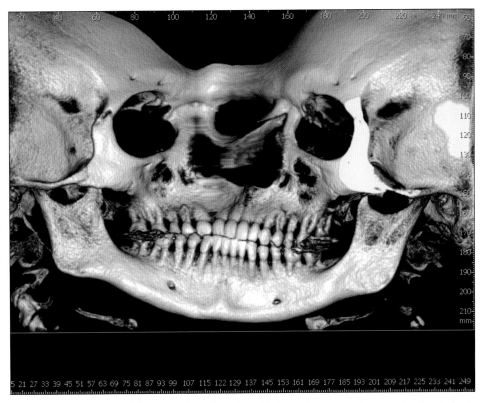

Fig 10-1b The shortened right ramus is confirmed on this 3-D color panoramic reconstruction. A shortened condylar neck is also visualized.

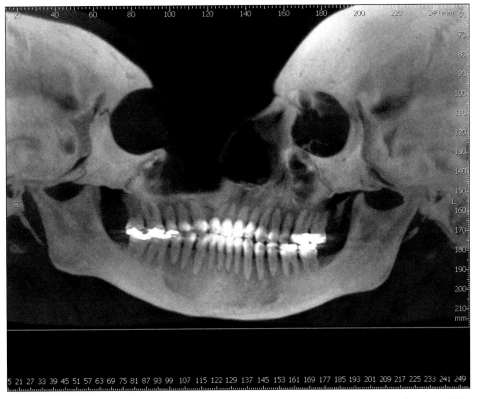

Fig 10-1c A maximum intensity projection (MIP) image of the panoramic reconstruction from Fig 10-1b. The distorted image of the cranium is due to the large-volume machine data.

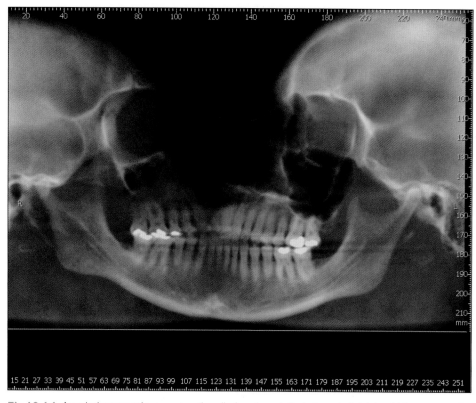

Fig 10-1d A typical panoramic reconstruction displays the calcified, elongated stylohyoid ligament on the patient's right side. This can also be seen in the 3-D color panoramic reconstruction in Fig 10-1b. This image shows the shorter right ramus as part of the facial asymmetry, but it is much less graphic than in Fig 10-1b.

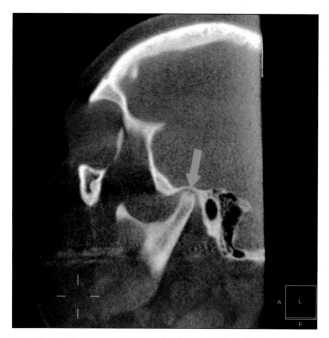

Fig 10-1e During radiologic evaluation, a subchondral cyst and subchondral sclerosis were discovered on the left condylar head *(arrow)*. This finding could impact the outcome of the proposed orthognathic surgery.

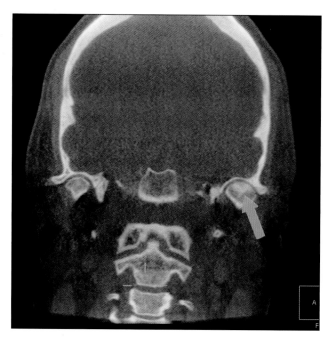

Fig 10-1f A coronal section from the data volume confirms the condylar changes.

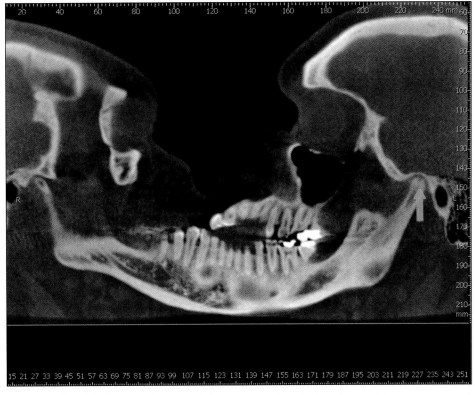

Fig 10-1g The thin slice pseudopanoramic image also confirms the condylar cyst *(arrow)*. This was *not* visualized on the panoramic reconstruction.

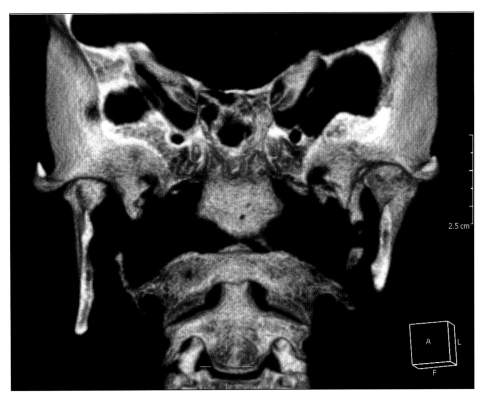

Fig 10-1h This 3-D color reconstruction (20 mm) best reveals the hypoplastic right condyle and neck, yet another component contributing to the facial asymmetry.

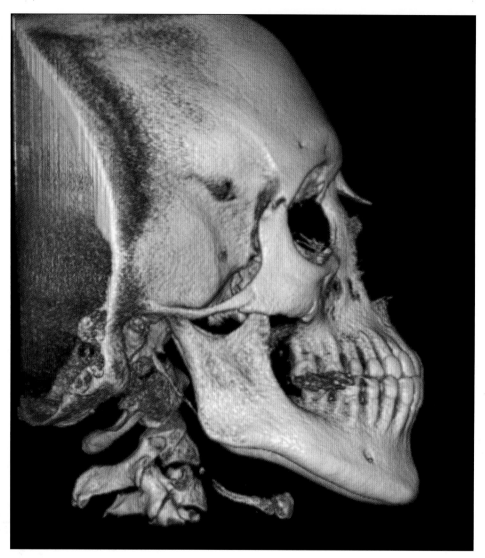

Fig 10-1i Preoperative view of the patient's right side.

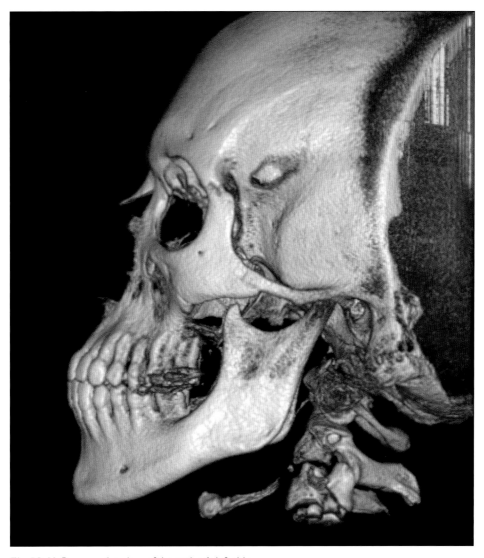

Fig 10-1j Preoperative view of the patient's left side.

FIG
10-2

MANDIBULAR FRACTURE: PREOPERATIVE
EVALUATION

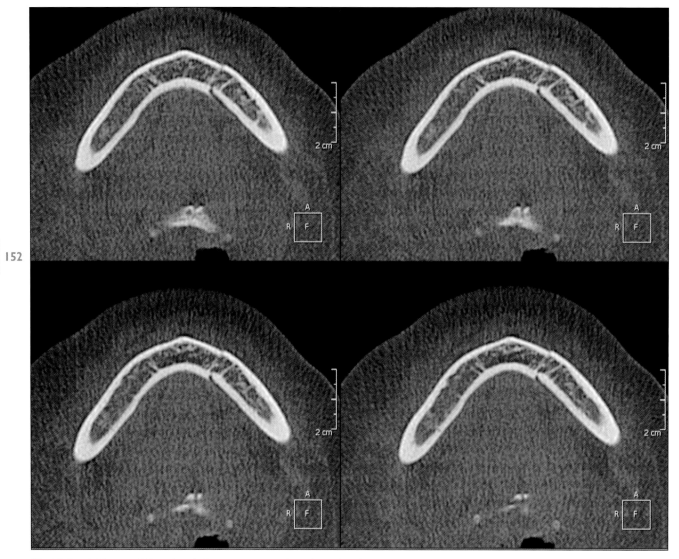

Fig 10-2a A 32-year-old American Indian woman was referred to an imaging center at an oral and maxillofacial surgeon's office in South Dakota for evaluation of a suspected mandibular fracture. These slices show a left-side anterior mandibular fracture with slight displacement of the fragments.

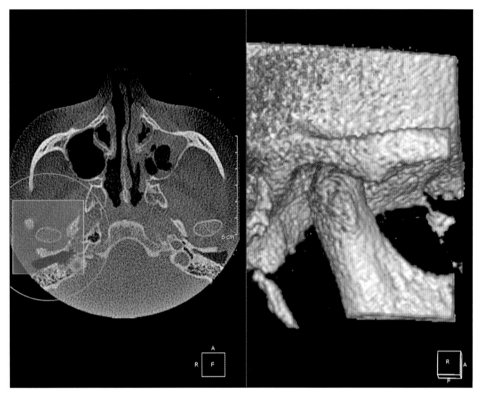

Fig 10-2b A reconstruction of the patient's right condyle from the lateral view shows no fracture present.

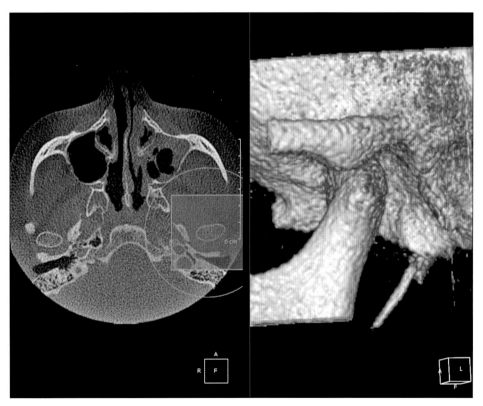

Fig 10-2c A reconstruction of the patient's left condyle from the lateral view shows no fracture present.

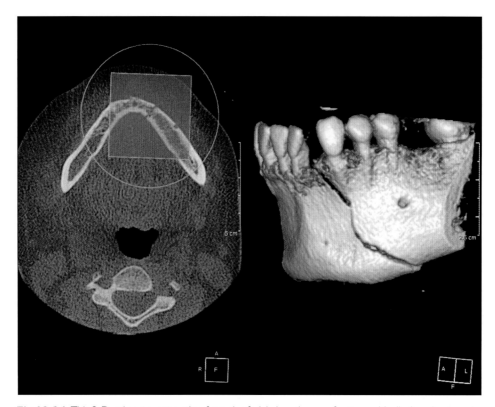

Fig 10-2d This 3-D color reconstruction from the facial view shows a fracture with displaced segments.

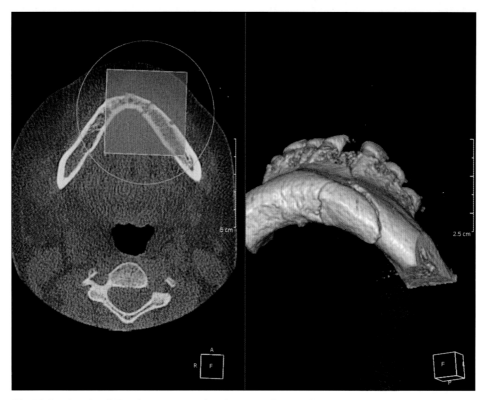

Fig 10-2e Another 3-D color reconstruction shows the fracture from the inferior view. Note the second fracture line nearer to the midline.

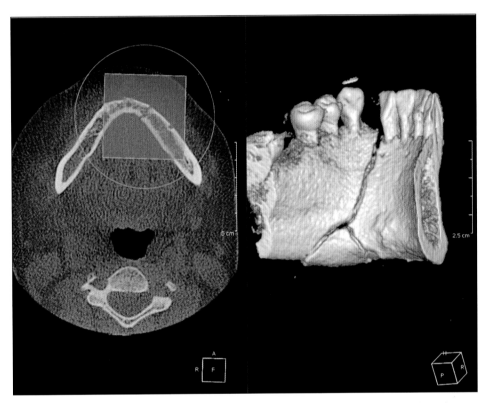

Fig 10-2f A third 3-D color reconstruction shows the fracture from the lingual aspect. Here, the true extent of the lower portion of the fracture can be appreciated.

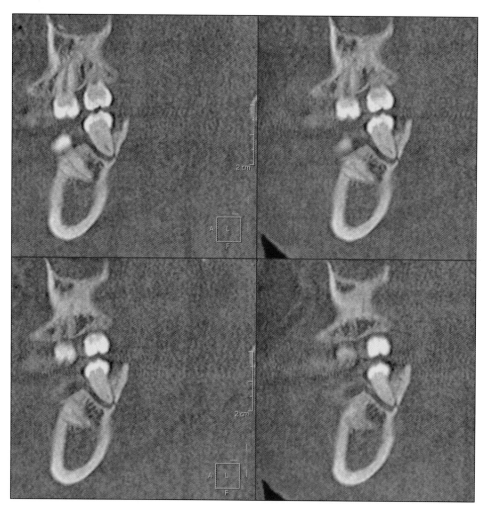

Fig 10-2g Another fracture, located more posteriorly on the right side, has caused the tooth to dislodge.

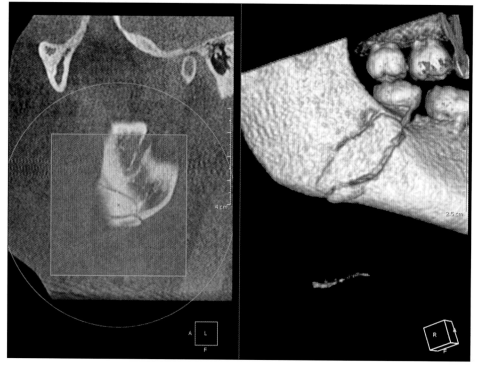

Fig 10-2h A 3-D color reconstruction shows the fracture from the facial view in the second molar region. This fracture apparently extends through the tooth socket.

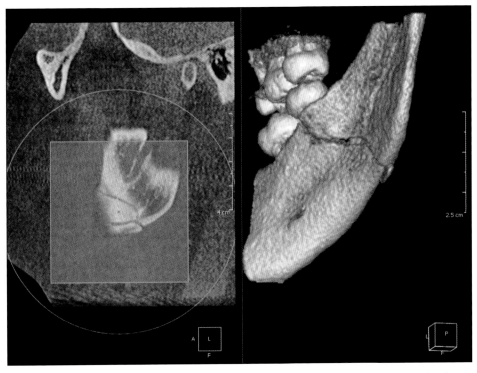

Fig 10-2i A 3-D color reconstruction shows the fracture from a posterior view in the second molar region. This fracture extends through the inferior mandibular border and submandibular fossa to the tooth socket.

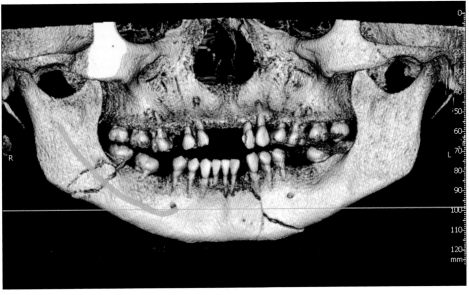

Fig 10-2j A 3-D color reconstruction shows the position of the inferior alveolar nerve (*orange line*) relative to the fracture lines.

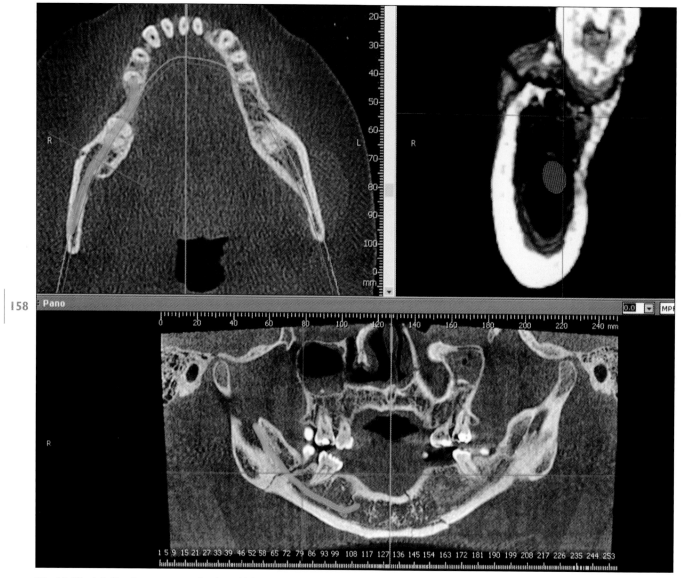

Fig 10-2k A 3-D color reconstruction in a thickened cross section *(top right)* shows the position of the inferior alveolar nerve *(red dot)* in relation to the second molar.

FIG

10-3

CHIN ADVANCEMENT: POSTOPERATIVE EVALUATION

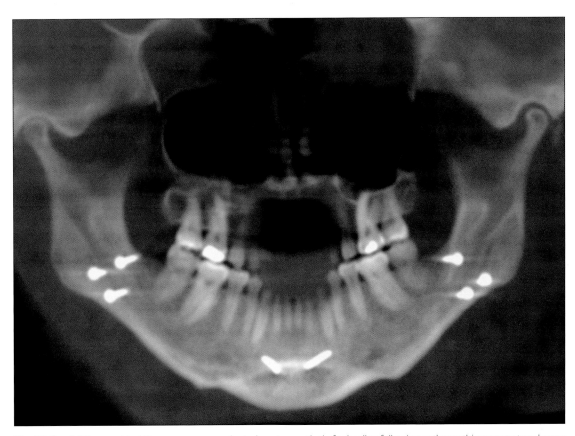

Fig 10-3a A 38-year-old white woman was evaluated postoperatively for healing following orthognathic surgery to advance her chin. This panoramic reconstruction shows the condylar positions and gross occlusal relationships. Note the discontinuity of the sections of the anterior mandible. Although this is an acceptable panoramic image, this particular reconstructed plane of section does not show the complete anterior maxilla.

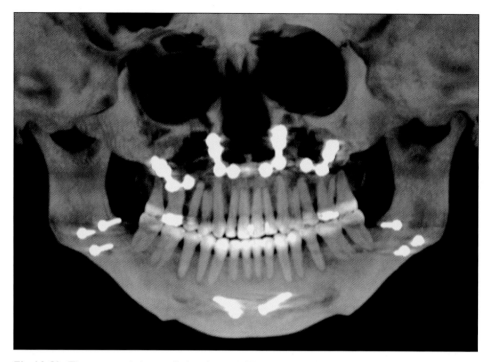

Fig 10-3b The panoramic image displayed as an MIP image shows more detail regarding the positions of the surgical plates and screws. The occlusion is shown more precisely, but the anterior mandible is somewhat distorted.

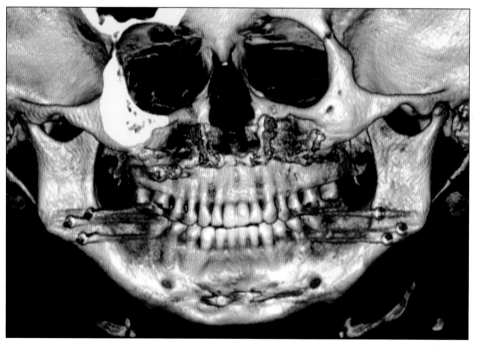

Fig 10-3c A 3-D color reconstruction in a panoramic mode details the exact appearance of the anatomic structures. Unfortunately, there are some scatter artifacts from the metallic objects. This reconstruction was done at a thickness of 30 mm. If a thicker slab rendering had been performed (at a thickness of 50 to 60 mm), then the right zygoma would have been displayed as nicely as the left.

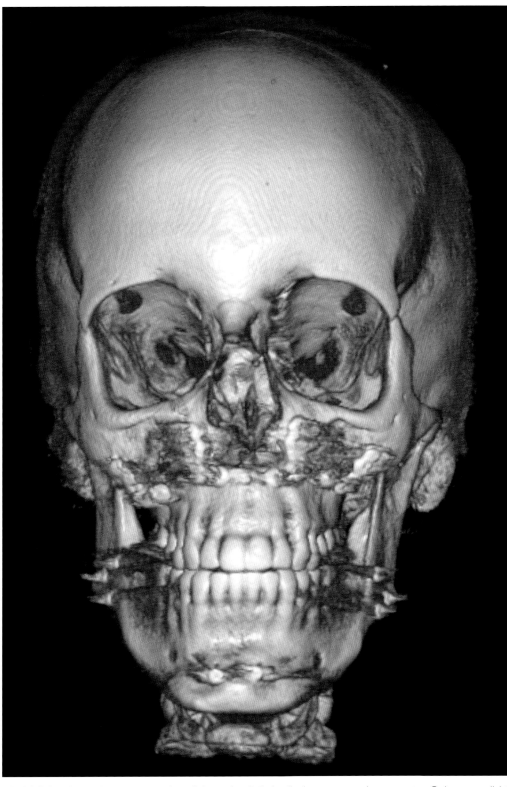

Fig 10-3d A 3-D color reconstruction of the entire skull details the postoperative symmetry. Only a very slight midline deviation remains.

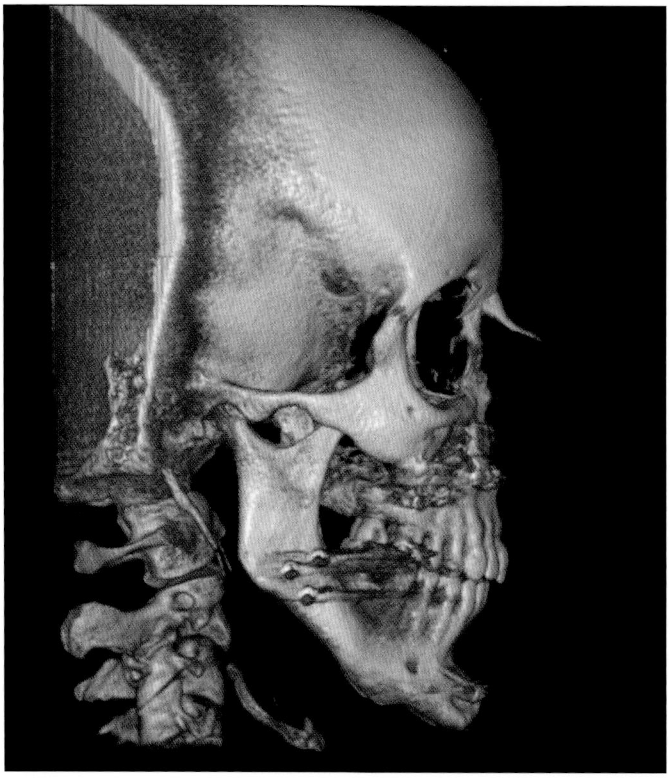

Fig 10-3e Right lateral view of the 3-D color reconstruction of the entire skull.

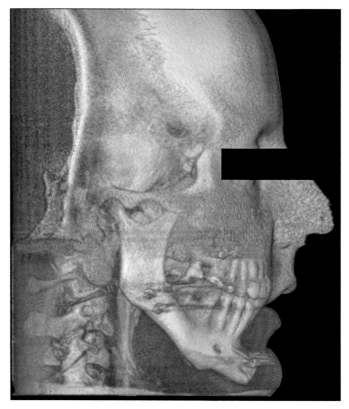

Fig 10-3f Right lateral view of the 3-D color reconstruction with transparent soft tissue overlay to reveal the final esthetic result.

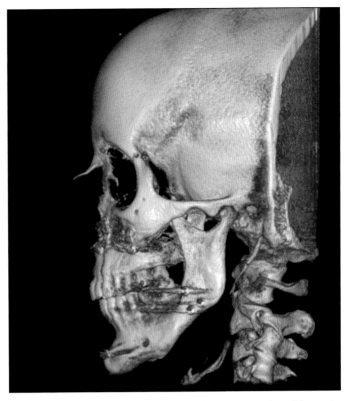

Fig 10-3g Left lateral view of the 3-D color reconstruction of the entire skull.

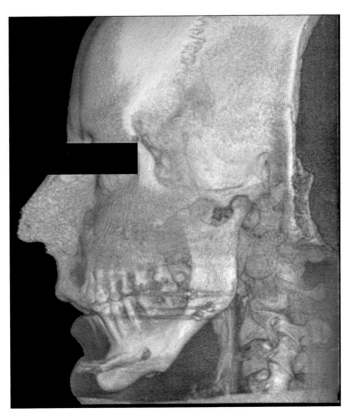

Fig 10-3h Left lateral view of the 3-D color reconstruction with transparent soft tissue overlay to reveal the final esthetic result.

Fig
10-4

Mandibular Advancement: Postoperative Evaluation

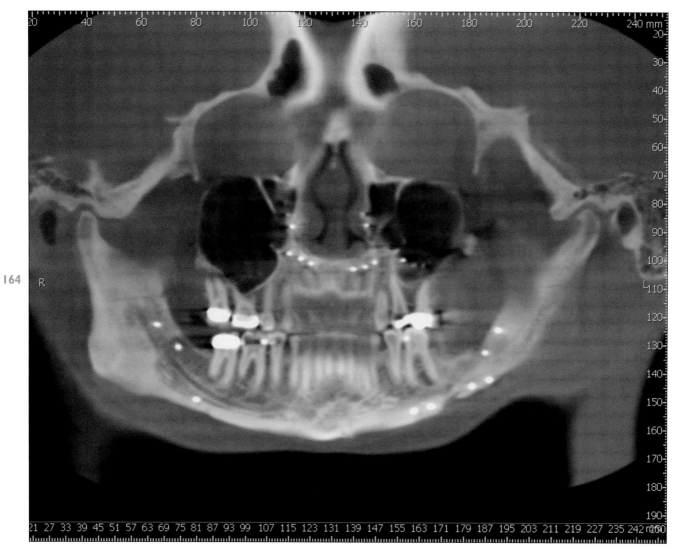

Fig 10-4a A white woman was referred to an imaging center for postoperative evaluation of a procedure to advance her entire mandible and correct a facial asymmetry. In this thin slice pseudopanoramic reconstruction showing the condyles, it is impossible to visualize the surgical devices completely.

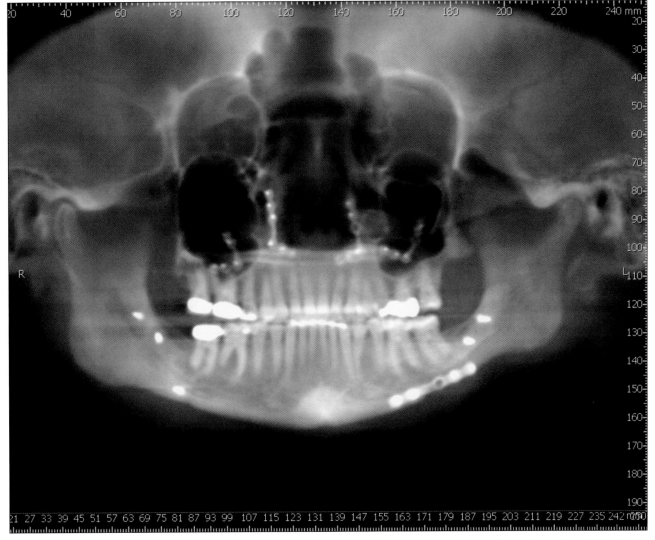

Fig 10-4b A panoramic view has been rendered in a thicker slice to see more detail. Now it is possible to discern the surgical stabilization bar in the left side of the mandible. Note that the left ramus appears to be much shorter than the right ramus.

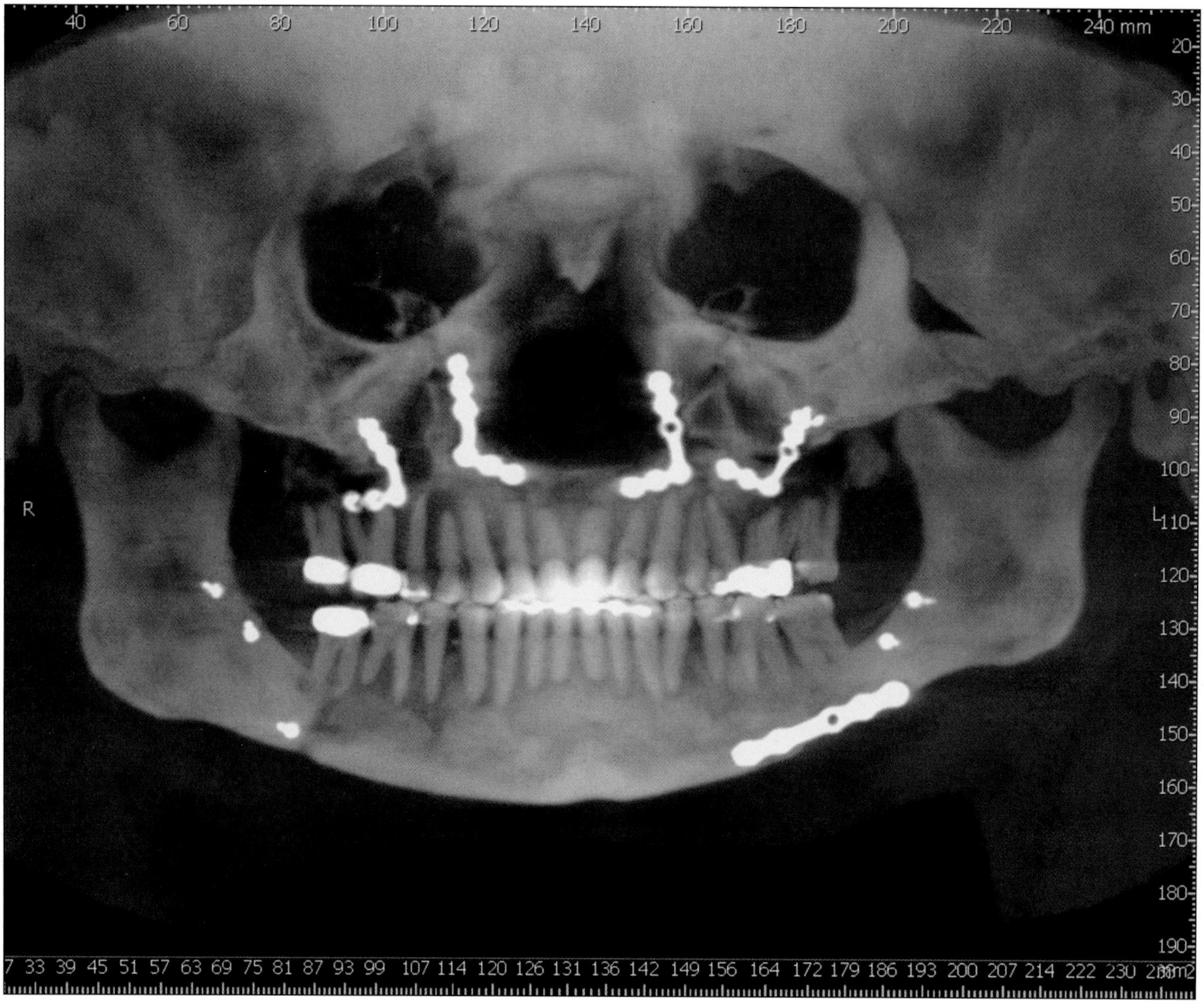

Fig 10-4c The MIP view shows occlusal detail and condylar fossa relationships. The bony asymmetry has improved substantially.

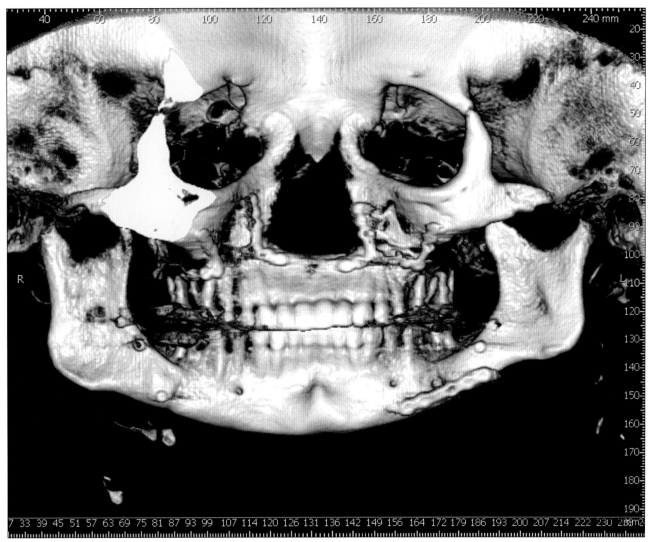

167

Fig 10-4d This 3-D color panoramic reconstruction emphasizes the symmetric result.

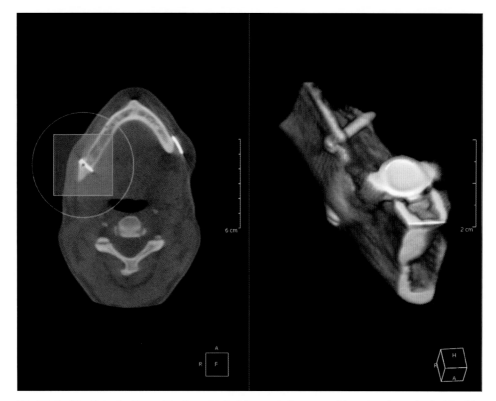

Fig 10-4e The Cube tool is used to show detail of the surgical screw positioned on the patient's right side.

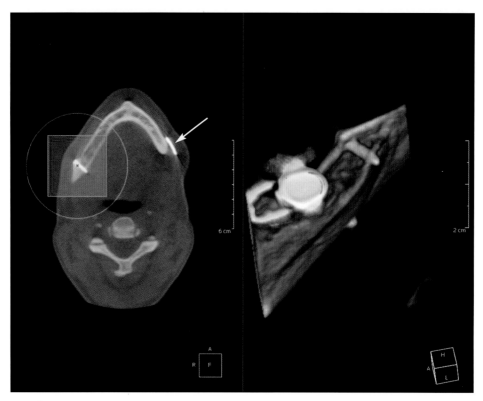

Fig 10-4f The surgical screw in Fig 10-4e is viewed from the lingual aspect. The position of the stabilization bar on the left side (*arrow*) starts to become visible as well.

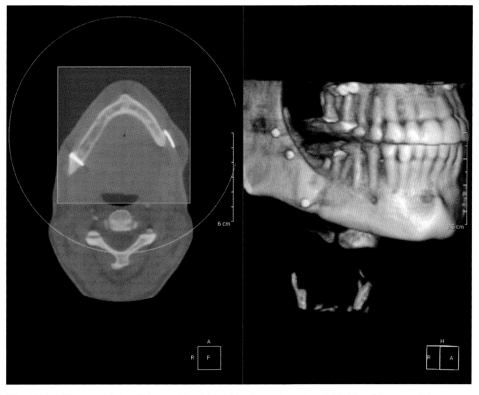

Fig 10-4g The area of the Cube tool is widened to show the entire right side of the mandible.

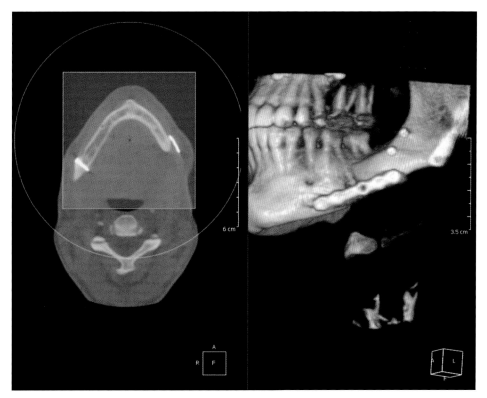

Fig 10-4h The area of the Cube tool is widened to show the entire left side of the mandible.

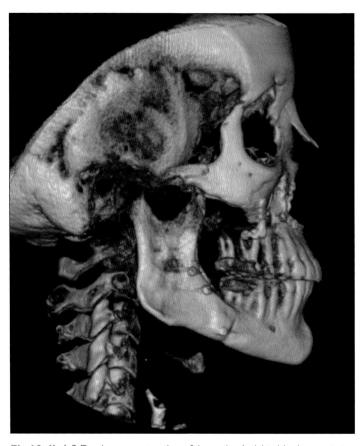

Fig 10-4i A 3-D color reconstruction of the patient's right side demonstrates the surgical outcome.

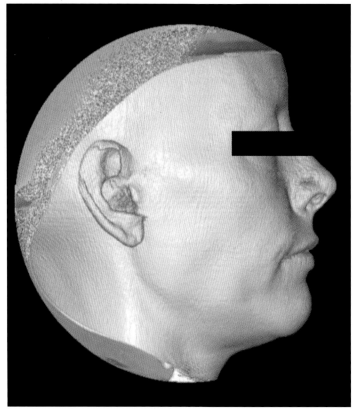

Fig 10-4j A soft tissue rendering of the patient's right side.

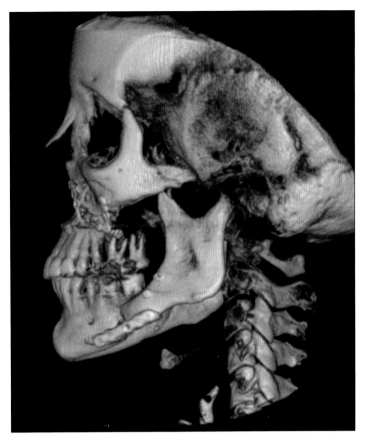

Fig 10-4k A 3-D color reconstruction demonstrates the surgical results on the patient's left side.

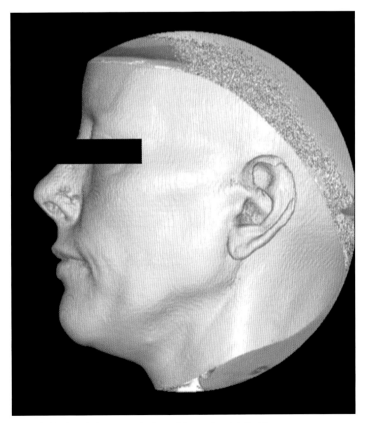

Fig 10-4l A soft tissue rendering of the patient's left side.

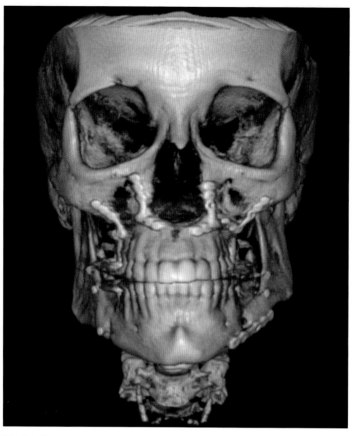

Fig 10-4m Note how the left mandibular angle flares out in this anteroposterior view.

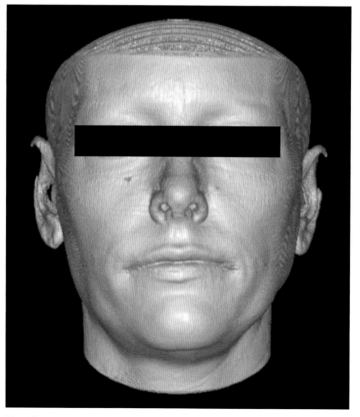

Fig 10-4n The soft tissue overlying the left mandibular angle in this rendering reveals a slight but acceptable asymmetry.

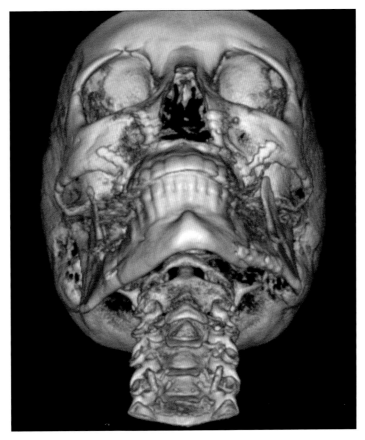

Fig 10-4o An image taken from Waters projection shows the bony structures of the patient.

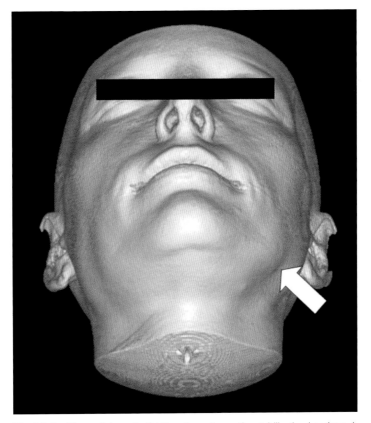

Fig 10-4p The soft tissue is slightly enlarged over the stabilization bar *(arrow)*.

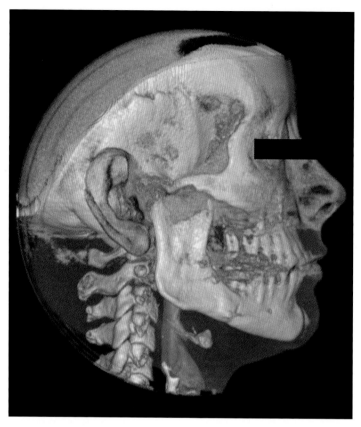

Fig 10-4q A right-side profile view of transparent soft tissue over bone reveals the surgical site.

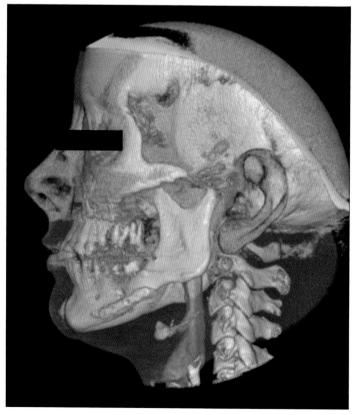

Fig 10-4r A transparent soft tissue profile on the left side also provides a view of the surgical site.

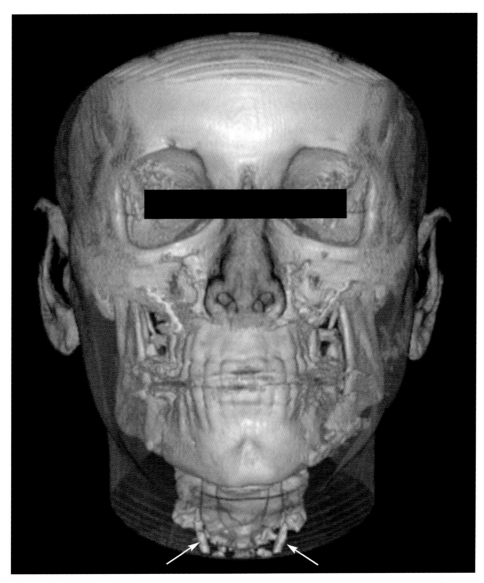

Fig 10-4s A transparent soft tissue anteroposterior view over bone shows the tracheal area. Note the calcification of the superior thyroid cartilage (arrows).

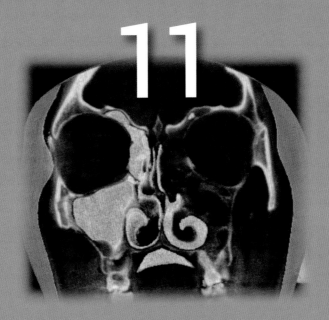

11

PARANASAL SINUS EVALUATION

Every dentist has treated a patient with toothache pain for which acute or chronic maxillary sinusitis is found to be the cause only after a thorough oral examination rules out an odontogenic origin. Furthermore, patients experiencing orofacial pain symptoms often require clinicians to evaluate headaches that may be caused by paranasal pathology. Even if the sinus involvement is suspected, how many times have clinicians underestimated a pansinusitis because only the maxillary sinuses could be imaged? Cone beam volumetric imaging (CBVI) is an exceptional way of imaging the paranasal sinus region in toto.

FIG

11-1

ROOT TIP AND ASSOCIATED INFLAMMATORY CHANGE

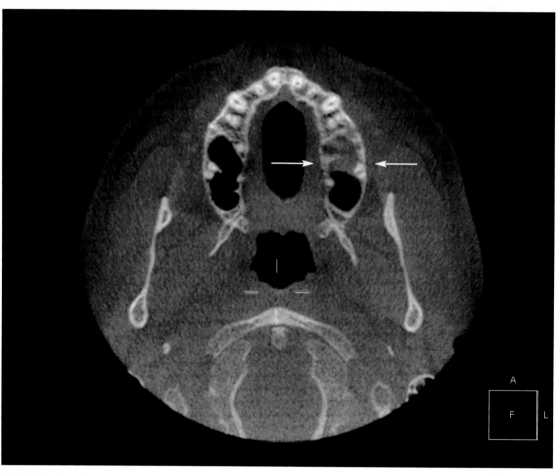

Fig 11-1a An axial section at the level of the maxillary first molar apices reveals an inflammatory change in the left antrum (*arrows*).

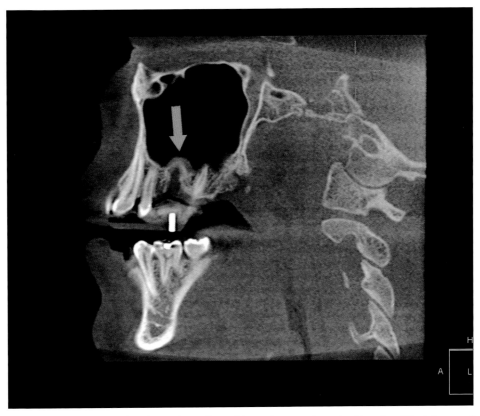

Fig 11-1b A sagittal section shows the radiographic marker over the extraction site of the left second premolar. Note the small uniform mucosal thickening over the apical area *(arrow)*.

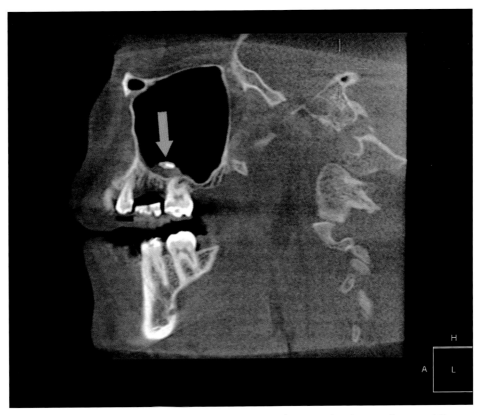

Fig 11-1c A sagittal section shows mucosal thickening over the extraction site, as well as a root tip containing endodontic fill material *(arrow)*.

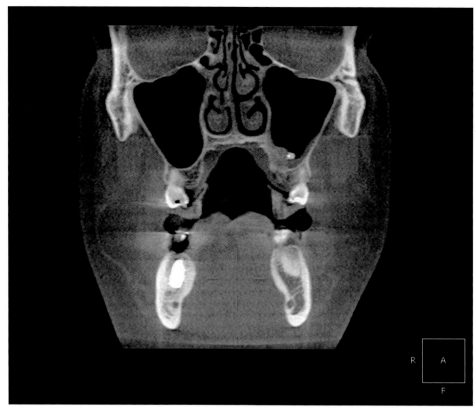

Fig 11-1d A coronal section shows mucosal thickening around the root tip. The root tip and fill material are just barely visible in this orientation.

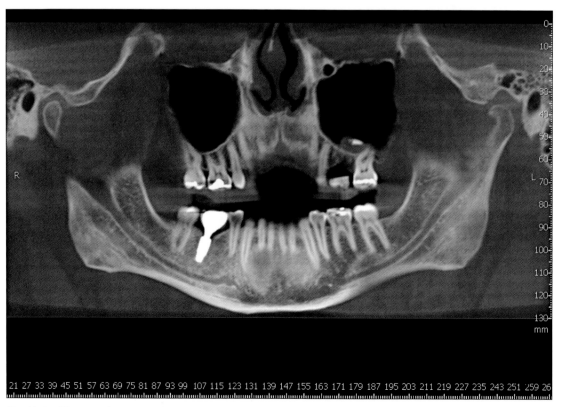

Fig 11-1e The root tip can be seen in this thin slice pseudopanoramic reconstruction.

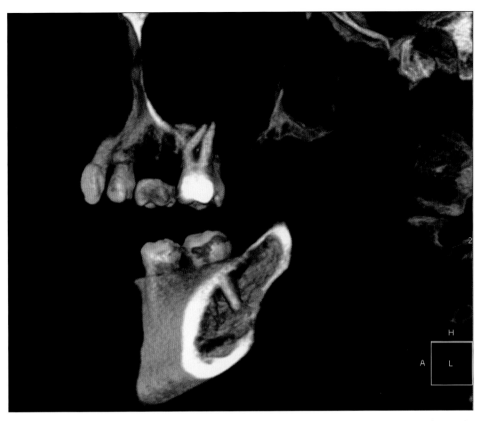

Fig 11-1f A 3-D color reconstruction shows the root tip of the first molar and its relation to the mesial root of the second molar.

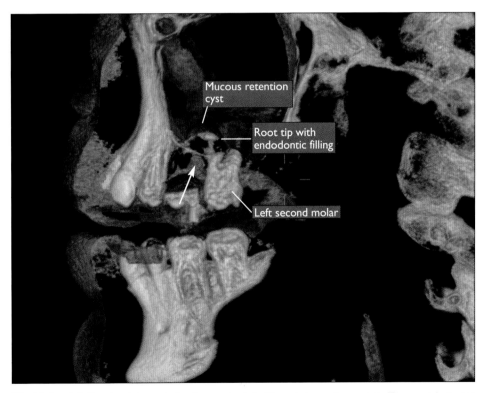

Fig 11-1g A 3-D color slab rendering (approximately 40 mm) shows the root tip. The space between the antral floor (arrow) and the root tip is where the inflammatory material would be. However, the margin of the reactive material can also be seen superior to the root tip of the extracted first molar as labeled.

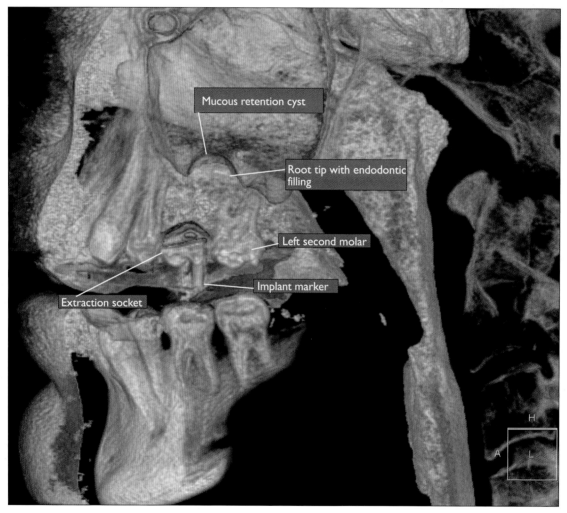

Fig 11-1h A 3-D color slab rendering (approximately 40 mm) shows the root tip of the first molar by using a Preset tool with different colors assigned to voxel transparency and opacity values.

Fig

11-2

MUCOUS RETENTION CYST

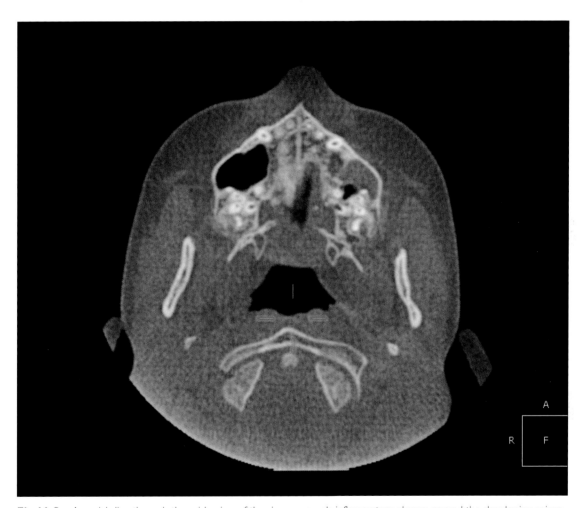

Fig 11-2a An axial slice through the midregion of the sinuses reveals inflammatory change around the developing apices.

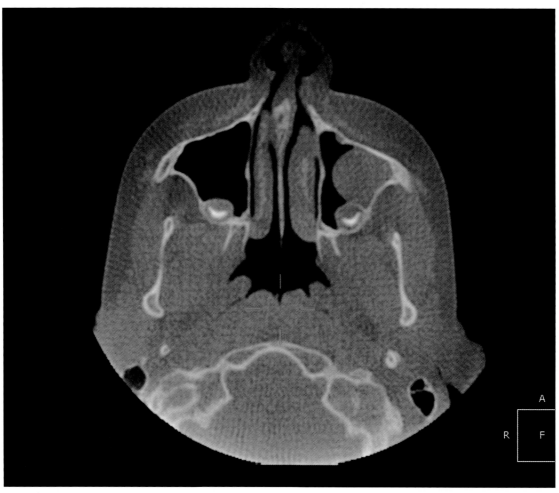

Fig 11-2b An axial slice through a more superior region of the antra shows the classic dome-shaped appearance of a mucous retention cyst, usually seen in a panoramic or lateral image.

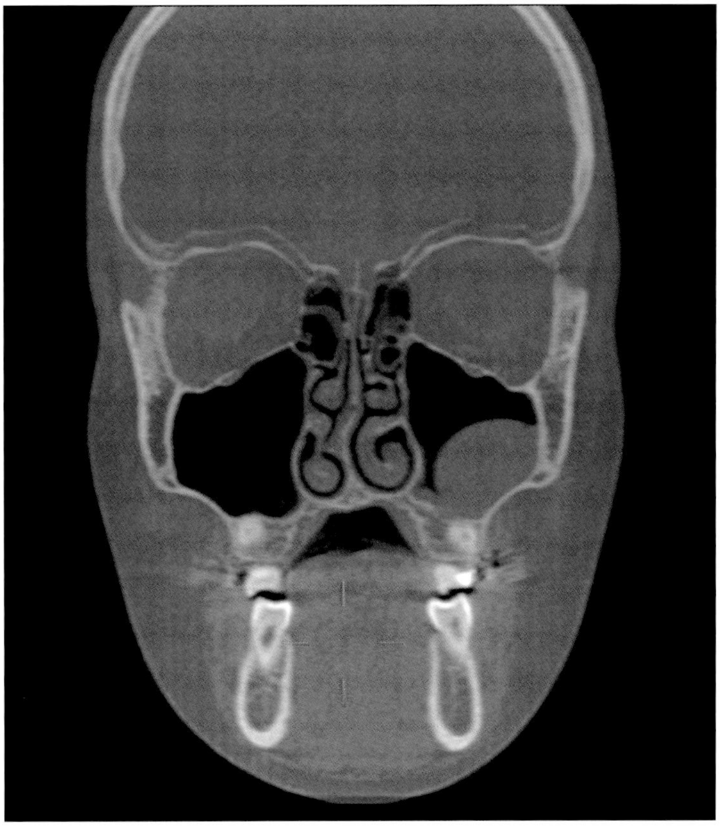

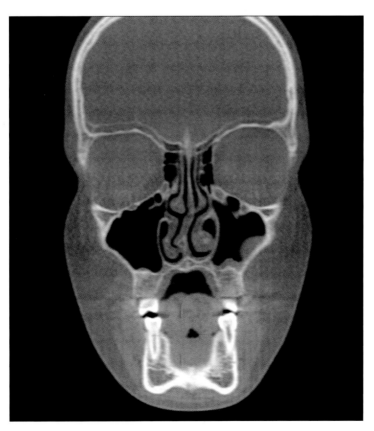

Fig 11-2c The dome shape of the mucous retention cyst is also visible arising from the floor of the left antrum in this coronal slice.

Fig 11-2d Another coronal slice shows the lesion getting smaller as the slice transsects a more posterior region of the antra.

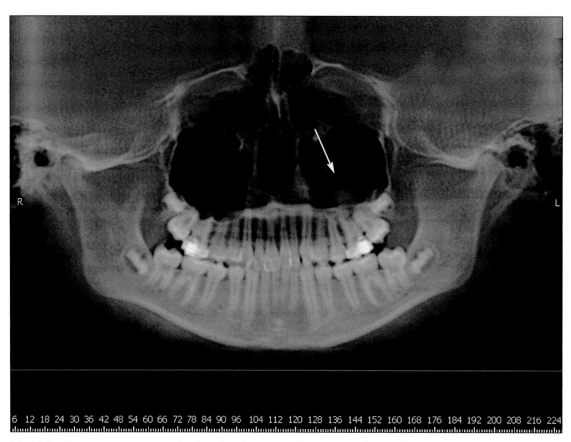

6 12 18 24 30 36 42 48 54 60 66 72 78 84 90 96 104 112 120 128 136 144 152 160 168 176 184 192 200 208 216 224

Fig 11-2e A panoramic reconstruction from the data volume demonstrates the usual appearance of a mucous retention cyst (*arrow*) seen in this mode.

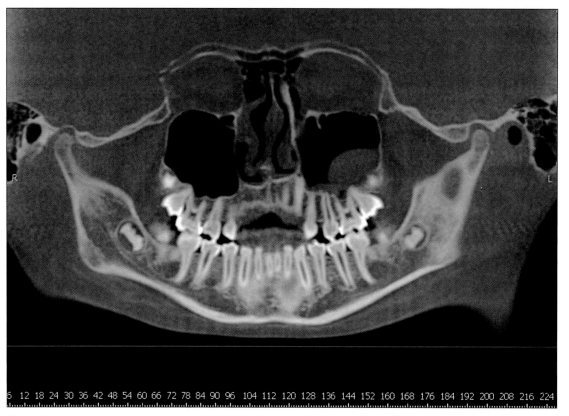

6 12 18 24 30 36 42 48 54 60 66 72 78 84 90 96 104 112 120 128 136 144 152 160 168 176 184 192 200 208 216 224

Fig 11-2f A pseudopanoramic reconstruction from the data volume shows the lesion more precisely because of the thin slice (0.15 mm) presentation.

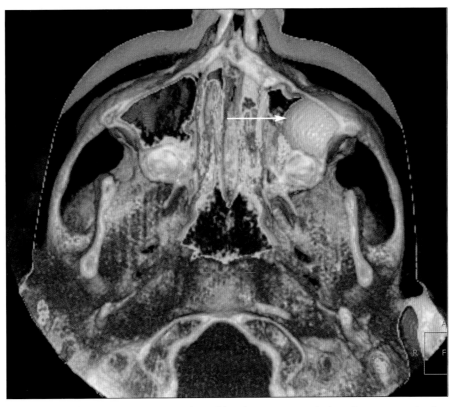

Fig 11-2g In this 3-D color reconstruction of the airway spaces, note how the mucous retention cyst has elevated the tissue of the left antrum *(arrow)*.

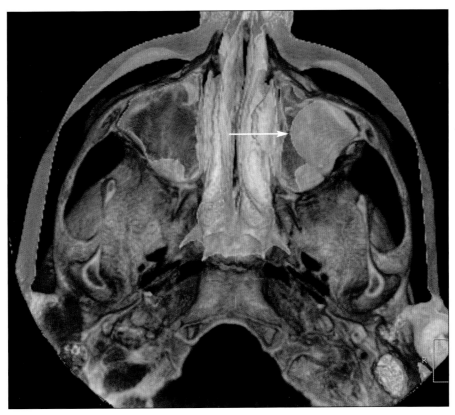

Fig 11-2h A different set of colors in a 3-D color reconstruction of the airway spaces shows the elevation of the tissue as transparent gray *(arrow)*.

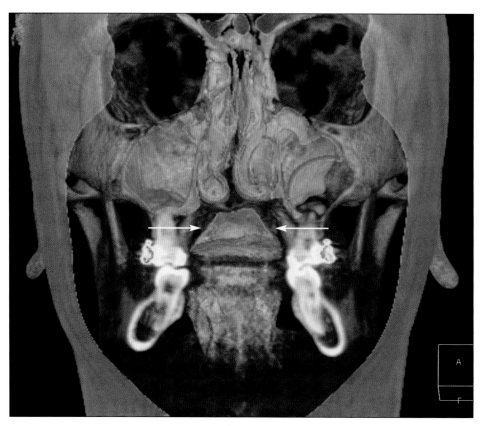

Fig 11-2i A coronal view of the same 3-D color reconstruction of the airway spaces and mucous retention cyst. The lesion border (an air–soft tissue interface) is seen distinctly as a darker gray line. The superior portion of the oropharyngeal airway is also well depicted (arrows).

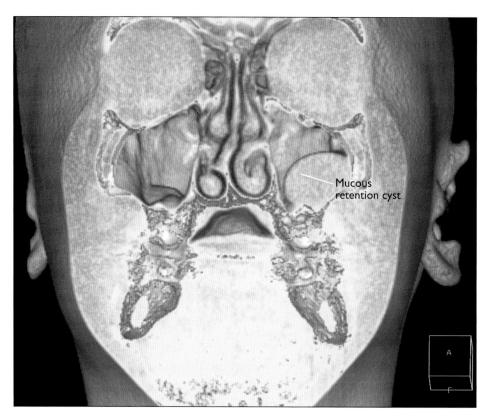

Mucous
retention cyst

Fig 11-2j A 3-D surface rendering has been cut away to show the mucous retention cyst.

FIG
11-3

PANSINUSITIS

Fig 11-3a A 9-year-old white girl was referred to an imaging service for evaluation of her permanent successor teeth. In this patient, almost all of the paranasal sinuses are opacified and filled with inflammatory product. An axial slice at the midregion of the condyle shows complete bilateral opacification of the antra. Note the early development of the permanent second molar follicles.

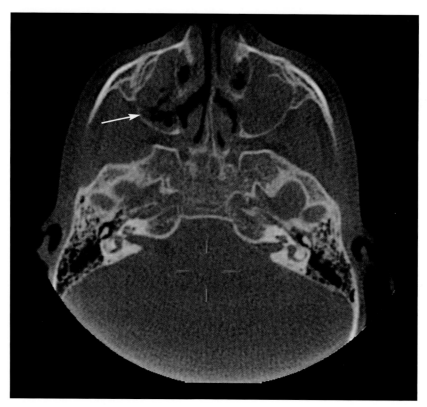

Fig 11-3b An axial slice above the condylar region shows complete opacification of the left antrum and mucous or air bubbles in a portion of the right antrum *(arrow)*.

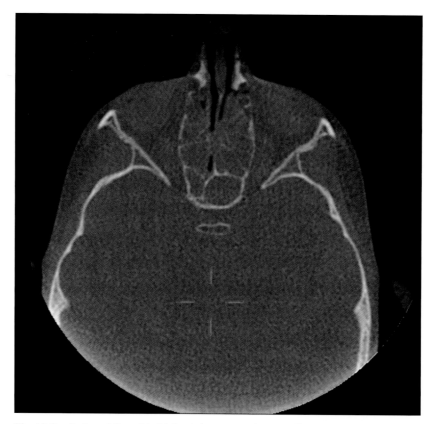

Fig 11-3c A slice at the midorbit level shows complete opacification of the ethmoid cell complex. The eyeballs and the optic nerves are visible through careful analysis.

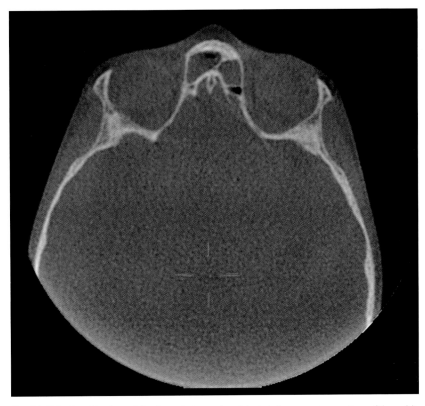

Fig 11-3d Opacification of the frontal sinuses is evident at the superior portion of the orbit.

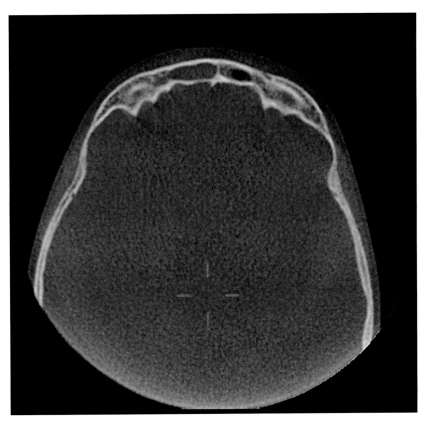

Fig 11-3e Opacification of the right frontal sinus and most of the left is seen in the inferior region of the orbit.

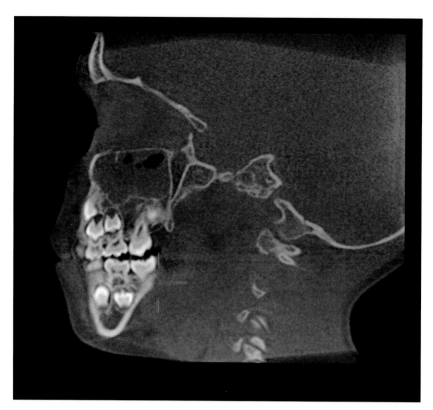

Fig 11-3f A sagittal view of the opacification of the left maxillary sinus confirms the presence of air bubbles.

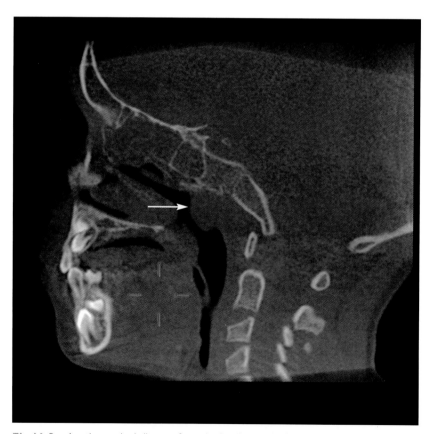

Fig 11-3g Another sagittal slice confirms the involvement of the ethmoid cells and an extension of the inflammatory change into the frontal sinus. The patient's adenoid tissues are also enlarged (arrow).

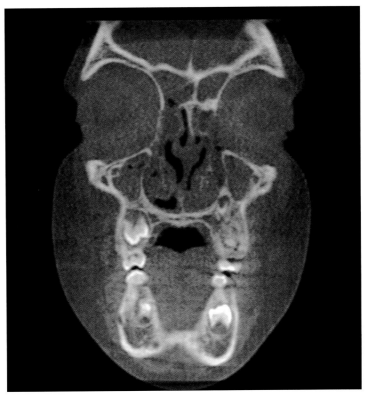

Fig 11-3h A coronal section of the maxillary antra, ethmoid cells, inferior nasal concha, osteomeatal complex, and frontal sinuses.

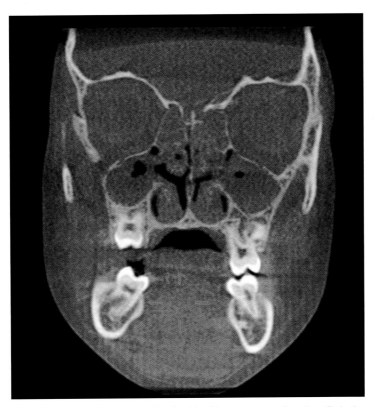

Fig 11-3i Similar regions are involved in this more posterior slice. Only the frontal sinuses are not seen here (compare to Fig 11-3h).

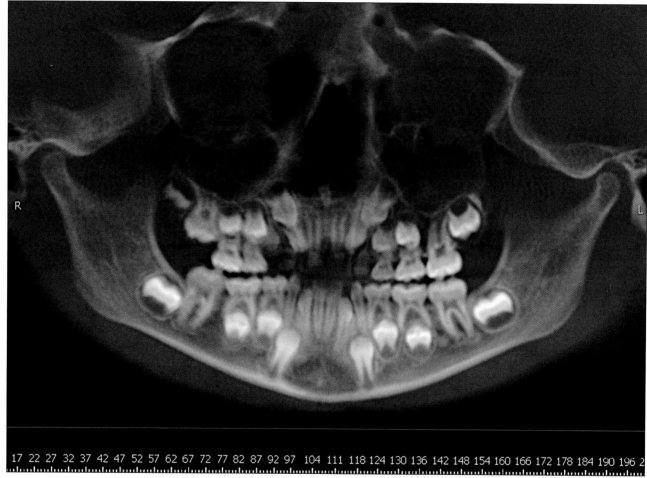

17 22 27 32 37 42 47 52 57 62 67 72 77 82 87 92 97 104 111 118 124 130 136 142 148 154 160 166 172 178 184 190 196 2

Fig 11-3j Although the maxillary sinus involvement is apparent in this typical panoramic view, the other airspace involvement would be grossly underestimated if this view alone were used for sinus evaluation.

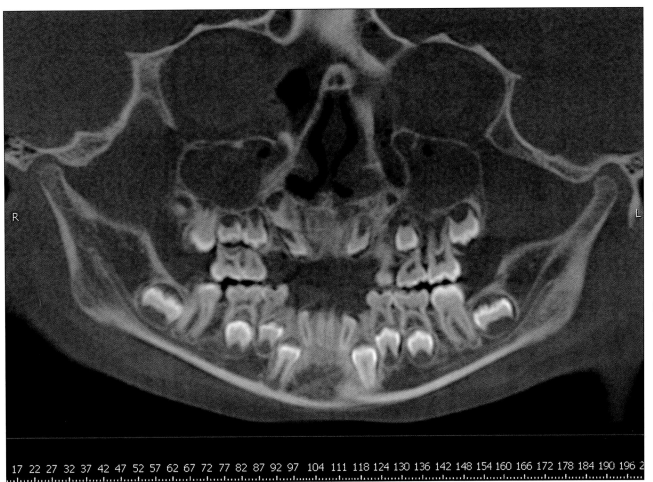

17 22 27 32 37 42 47 52 57 62 67 72 77 82 87 92 97 104 111 118 124 130 136 142 148 154 160 166 172 178 184 190 196 2

Fig 11-3k This thin slice pseudopanoramic reconstruction is only slightly better at demonstrating the involvement of the paranasal sinuses.

FIG

11-4

ETHMOID LESION

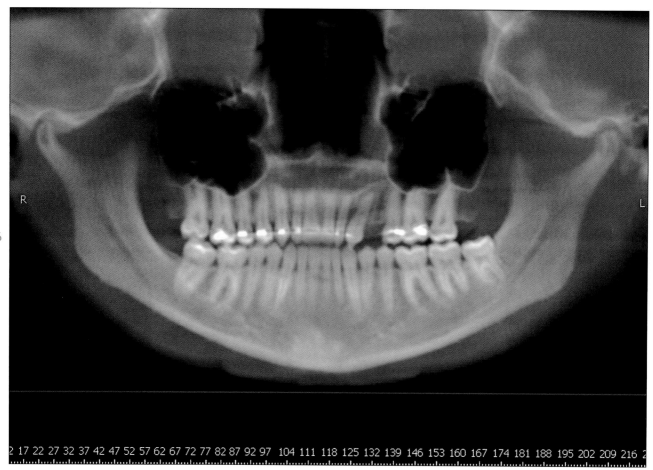

Fig 11-4a A 27-year-old white man was referred to an imaging service for an orthodontic evaluation during treatment to assess the maxillary left canine after traction. In a panoramic reconstruction of the patient data volume, there is *no indication* of a problem in any of the visible paranasal or nasal spaces.

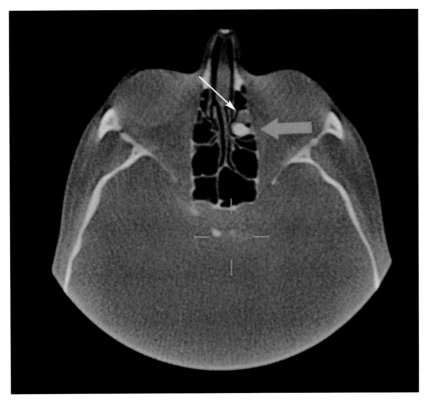

Fig 11-4b A solid radiopacity is seen in a left ethmoid cell *(blue arrow)* with inflammatory change (opacification) visible in an adjacent air cell *(white arrow)*.

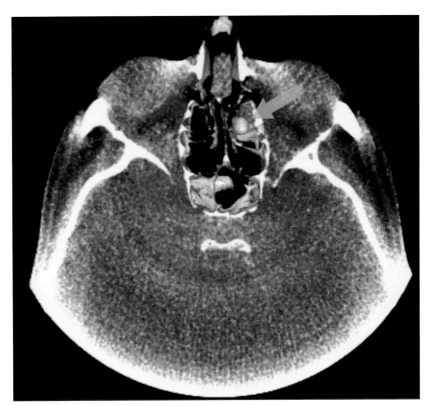

Fig 11-4c The same radiopacity seen in the left ethmoid cell *(blue arrow)* in a 3-D color slab rendering.

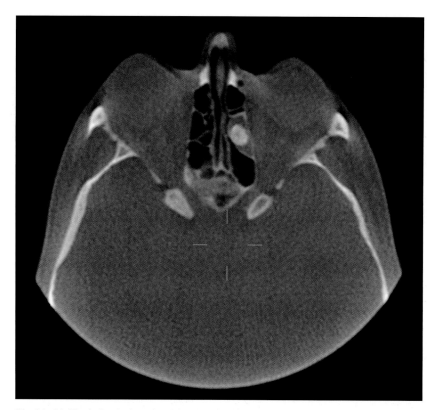

Fig 11-4d The lesion in the ethmoid region is an incidental finding. The solid radiopacity seen in Fig 11-4b has inflammatory change surrounding the lesion. The optic nerve and medial and lateral rectus muscles can also be seen faintly.

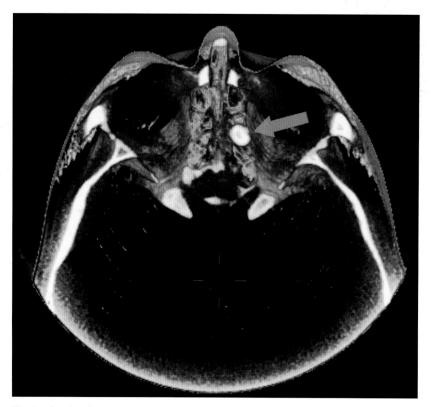

Fig 11-4e A different color rendering also shows this solid radiopacity in the left ethmoid cell (*blue arrow*).

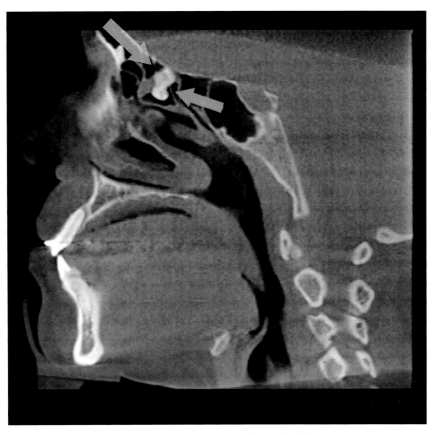

Fig 11-4f The ethmoid lesion *(arrows)* is highlighted in a sagittal view.

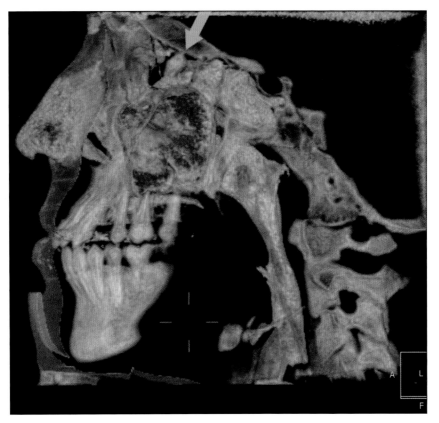

Fig 11-4g In this sagittal view of the ethmoid lesion *(arrow)*, the airway is colorized and an outline of the transparent soft tissue is provided.

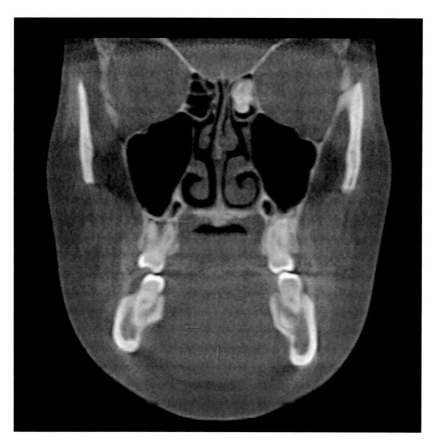

Fig 11-4h A thin coronal slice (0.15 mm) at the midregion of the sinus shows ethmoid cell opacity.

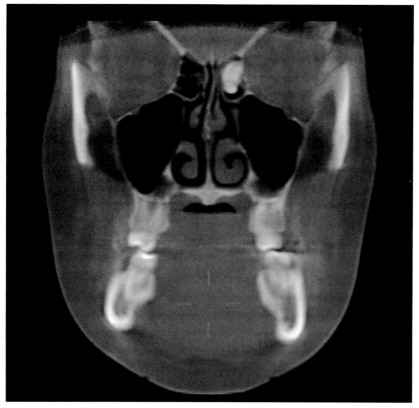

Fig 11-4i A thicker coronal slice (4.1 mm) at the same region also shows ethmoid cell opacity.

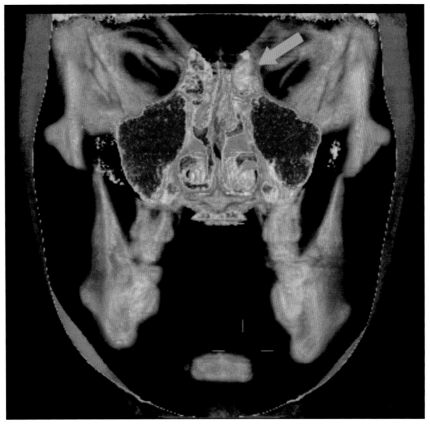

Fig 11-4j A colorized slab rendering of the ethmoid lesion *(blue arrow)* allows comparison of the left-side ethmoid lesion to the normal right-side ethmoid cells.

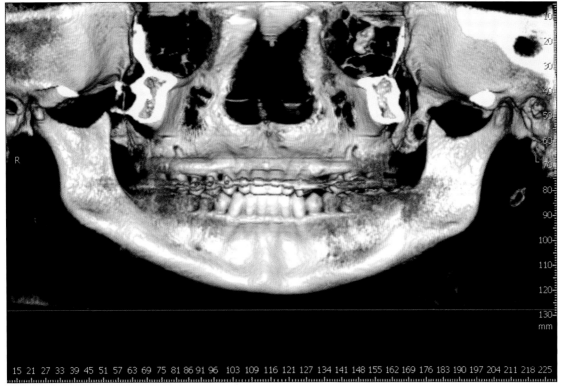

Fig 11-4k Unlike the more traditional panoramic image seen in Fig 11-4a, this 3-D color panoramic reconstruction *does* show the ethmoid lesion. Osteoma of the ethmoid bone has been reported only rarely.[1]

FIG
11-5

EXTRINSIC ANTRAL TUMOR

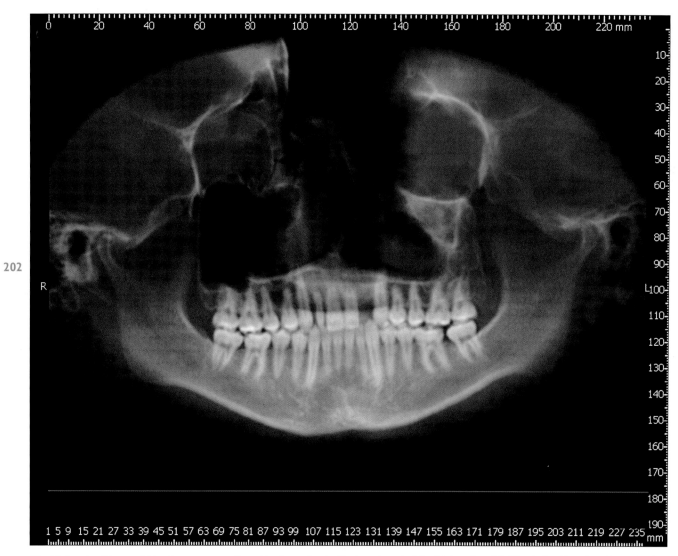

Fig 11-5a An 18-year-old Iranian man was referred to the orthodontic department at the University of California, San Francisco, for evaluation of a potential sinus problem. An extrinsic odontogenic tumor had invaded the left antrum secondarily.

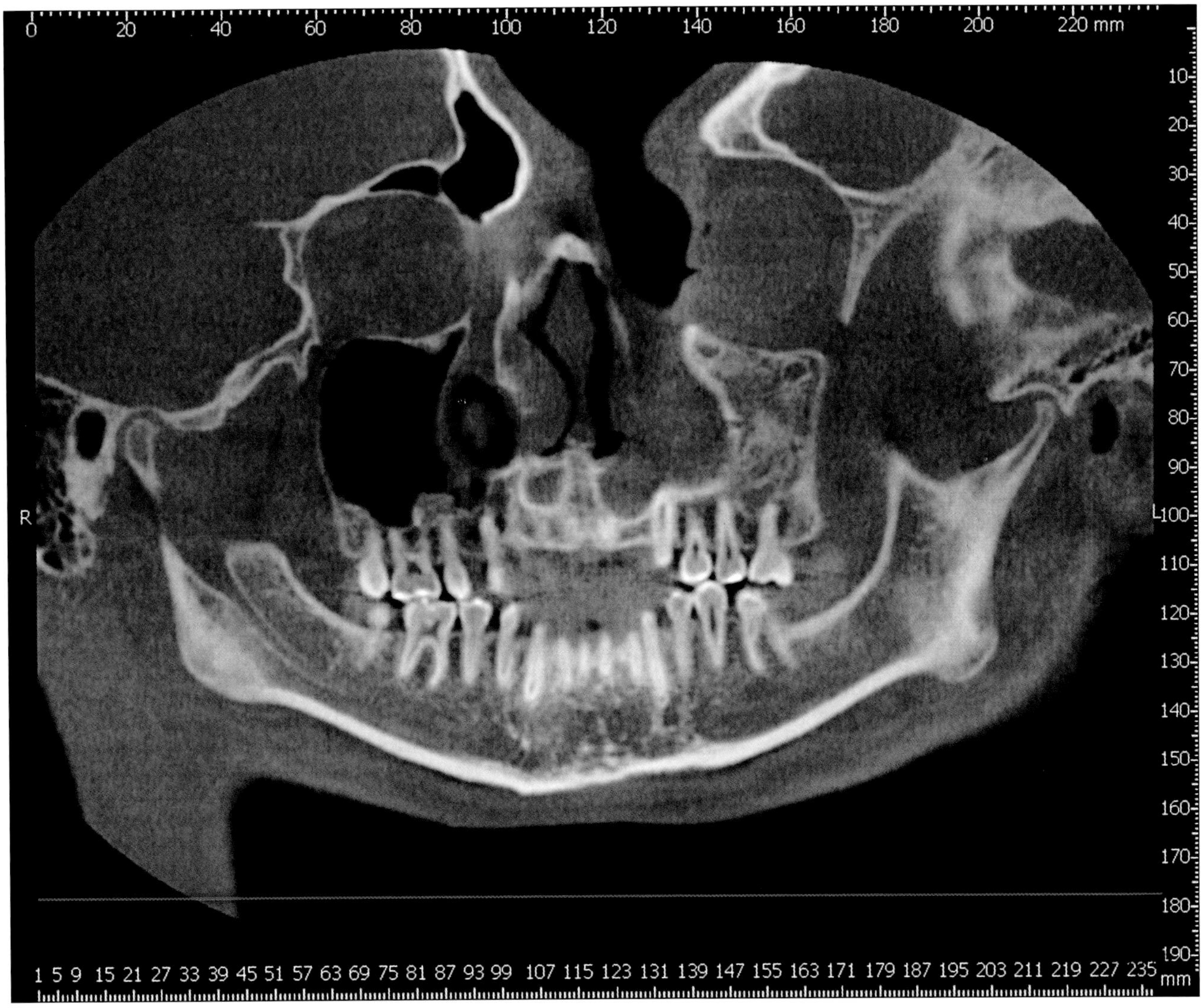

Fig 11-5b This thin slice pseudopanoramic reconstruction provides a clearer picture of the left antrum and nasal cavity than does Fig 11-5a. On the left side, note the lack of sinus air space, the hypoplastic condyle, and the altered malar region.

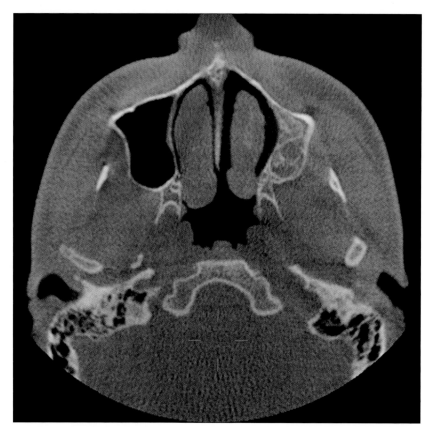

Fig 11-5c An axial slice shows the complete absence of the left sinus and replacement by a somewhat multilocular lesion.

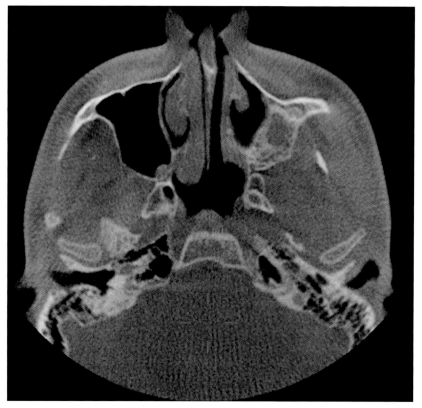

Fig 11-5d An axial slice at a slightly more superior level confirms that the lesion has replaced the antrum and extended into the malar region.

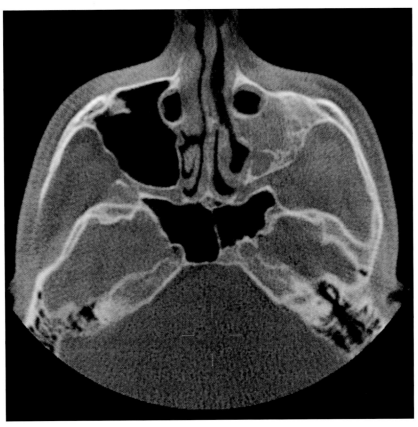

Fig 11-5e Another axial slice shows complete replacement of the left maxillary sinus, the multilocular appearance, and the suggestion of inflammatory product within the multilocular lesion itself.

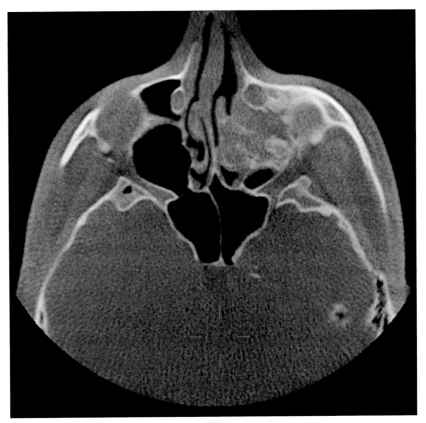

Fig 11-5f The lesion is shown extending into the middle meatal area and the ethmoid cells.

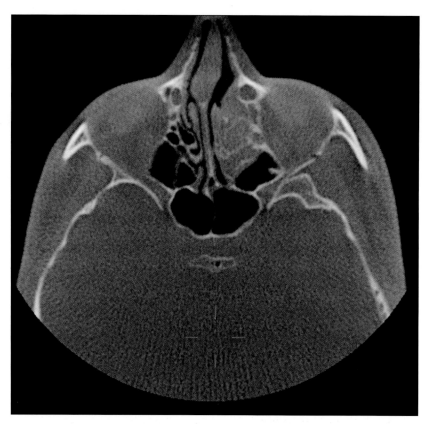

Fig 11-5g This slice reveals ethmoid cell involvement and possible displacement of the nasal septum to the right side.

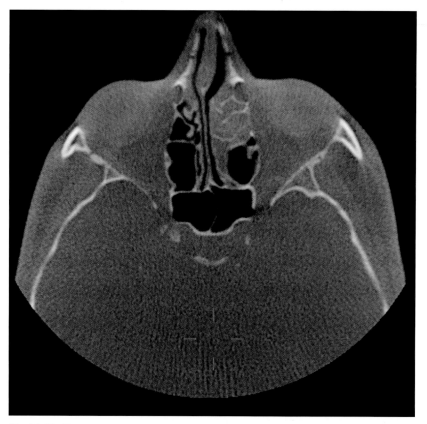

Fig 11-5h The lesion extends posteriorly into the ethmoid cells and has caused a loss of their normal architecture. The appearance is that of a multilocular lesion within the air cells.

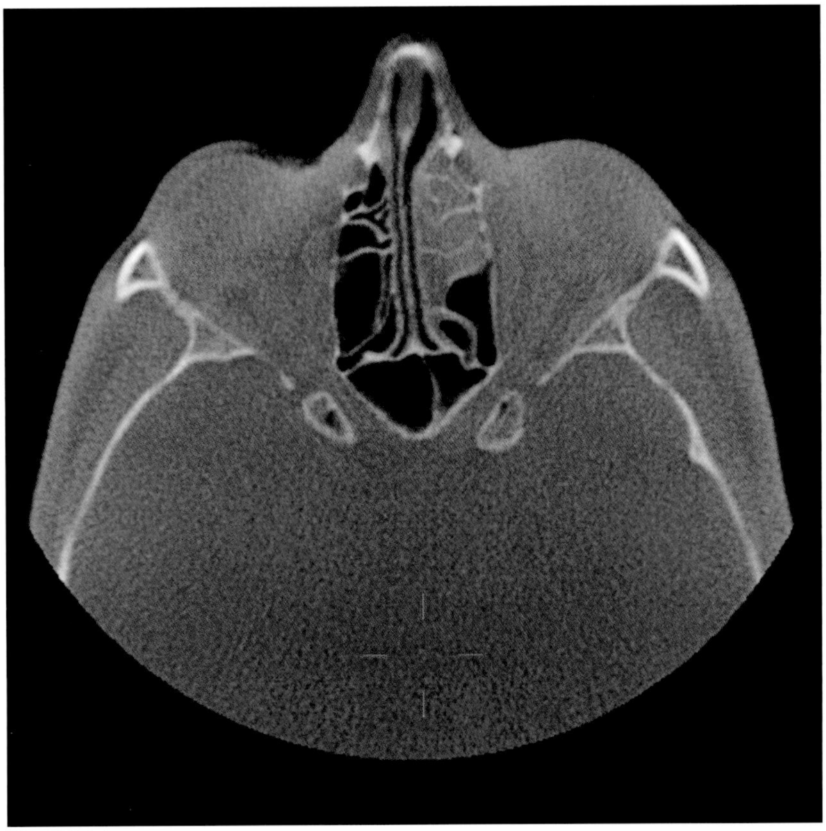

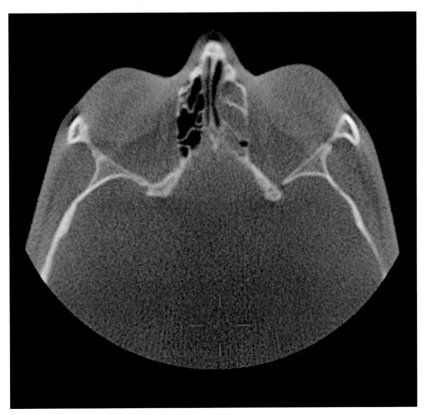

Fig 11-5i A slice demonstrating extension of the lesion into more air cells.

Fig 11-5j The lesion has reached the superior aspect of the ethmoid cell complex.

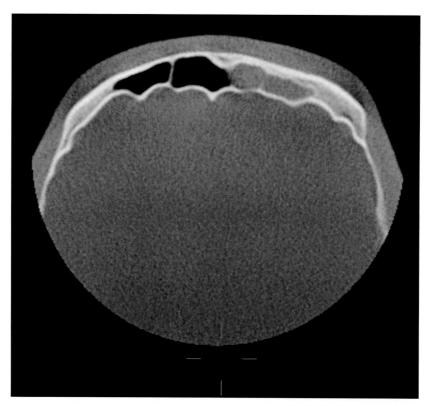

Fig 11-5k A more superior slice shows probable extension of the odontogenic lesion into the left frontal sinus.

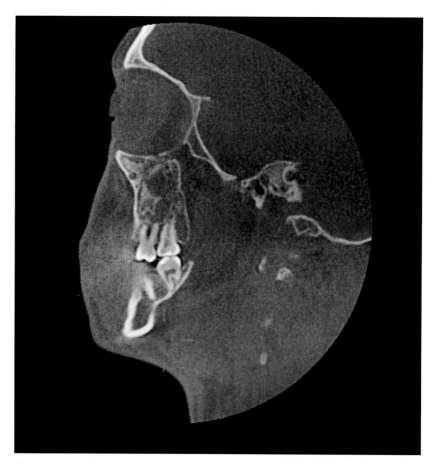

Fig 11-5l A sagittal view shows the lesion occupying the left side of the maxilla.

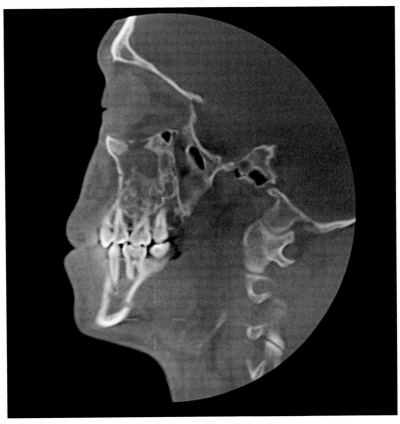

Fig 11-5m The multilocular appearance in this sagittal slice suggests loculi of variable size, which is most consistent with an ameloblastoma.

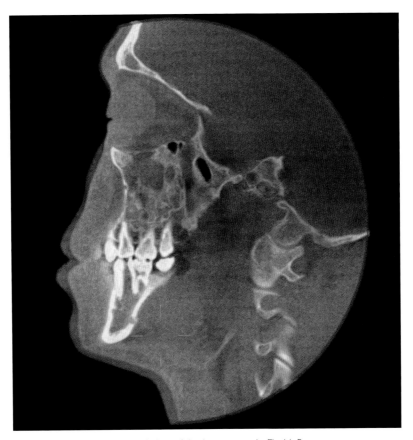

Fig 11-5n A 3-D color rendering of the image seen in Fig 11-5m.

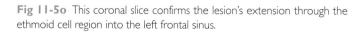

Fig 11-5o This coronal slice confirms the lesion's extension through the ethmoid cell region into the left frontal sinus.

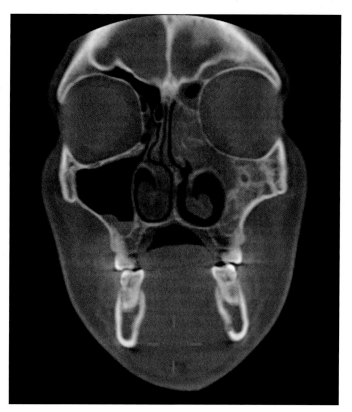

Fig 11-5p The frontal sinus opacification may just be secondary inflammatory change because of the blocked osteomeatal complex. Note the slight inflammatory change in the inferior region of the right antrum. Note also the enlarged right inferior meatus and deviation of the nasal septum.

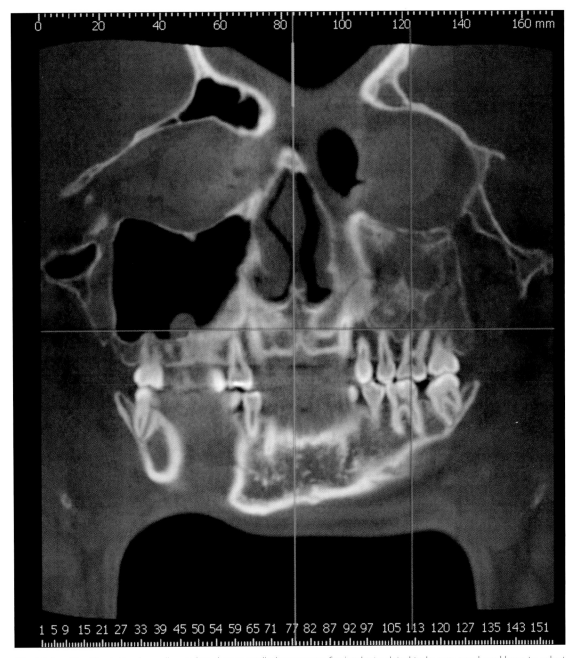

Fig 11-5q The Dental tool, usually used to draw a preliminary curve for implant-related tasks, was employed here to select a thin layer through the maxilla. This provides another look at the lesion characteristics visible in the left side of the maxilla.

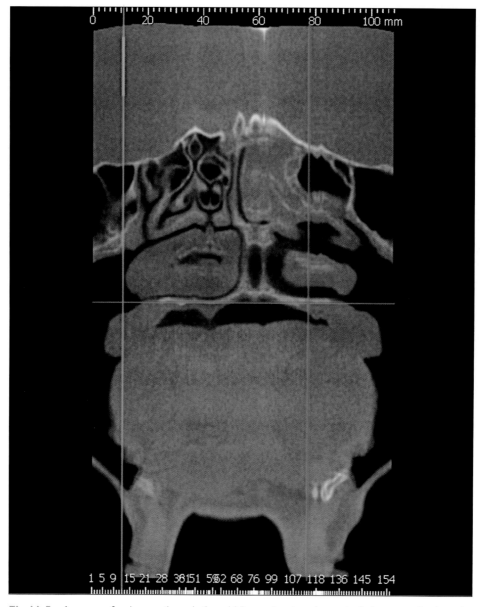

Fig 11-5r A more refined curve through the middle nasal region shows the lesion extension into the ethmoid cells.

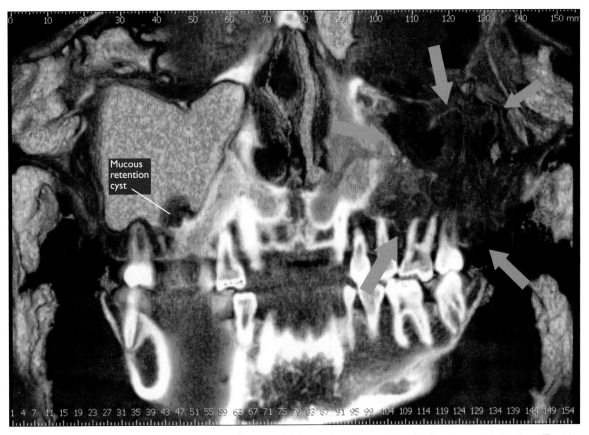

Fig 11-5s A 3-D color reconstruction compares the normal right maxillary sinus region with the abnormal left antrum. The *blue arrows* are an attempt to outline the margins of the lesion.

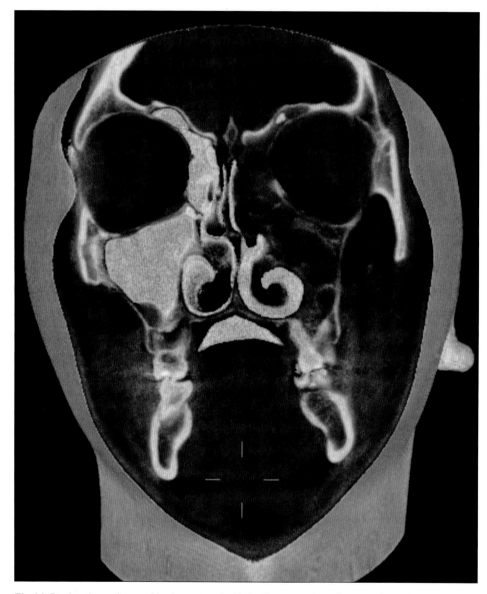

Fig 11-5t Another color combination created with the Presets tool confirms the area of the lesion from maxilla to frontal sinus.

REFERENCE

1. Lachanas VA, Koutsopoulos AV, Hajiioannou JK, Bizaki AJ, Helidonis ES, Bizakis JG. Osteoid osteoma of the ethmoid bone associated with dacryocystitis. Head Face Med 2006 Aug 4; 2:23.

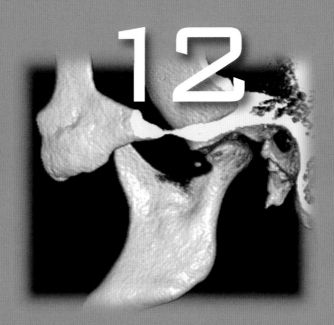

12

TEMPOROMANDIBULAR JOINT EVALUATION

One of the most fascinating applications of cone beam volumetric imaging (CBVI) for radiologists is the characterization of condylar changes and appearance of the temporomandibular joint (TMJ) complex. In conventional 2-D and tomographic imaging, dentists previously made assertions that a feature like the so-called bird-beak appearance was indicative of osteoarthritis or a loose body in the joint space (also known as a *joint mouse*). We used panoramic images as gross screening images, knowing that the image was not truly a lateral projection and therefore almost always underestimated the true changes. Several techniques were invented in an attempt to capture the condyle in its true position, or to slice up the condyle from medial to lateral pole to try to see the changes on various regions of the condylar head. As if it were not difficult enough to image the TMJ complex with conventional 2-D grayscale techniques, the variations in the condyle's shape and size from one side to the other made the task of interpreting significant changes even more challenging.

FIG
12-1

ALTERED CONDYLAR MORPHOLOGY

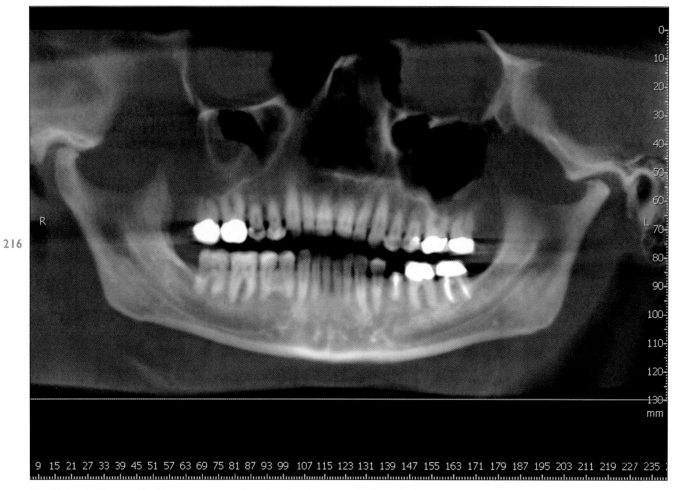

216

Fig 12-1a A 51-year-old white woman was referred to the Northwest Radiography imaging center in Bellevue, Washington, for evaluation of the TMJs after experiencing mild joint pain. A panoramic reconstruction shows a shortened left condylar neck and altered condylar morphology relative to the right condyle.

This kind of guesswork in radiographic interpretation will become a thing of the past with the use of CBVI. True condylar shapes in 3-D and color can replace the 2-D grayscale "Rorschach tests" we used for TMJ assessment. For all clinicians, this represents a huge leap in our understanding of the condyles, the TMJ complex, and the appearance of these structures in response to arthritic insults and systemic alterations.

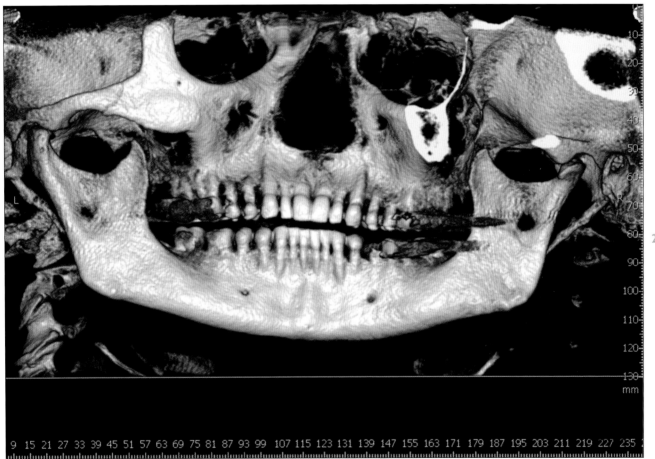

Fig 12-1b A 3-D color reconstruction of the panoramic radiograph in Fig 12-1a shows more detail of the clinical situation.

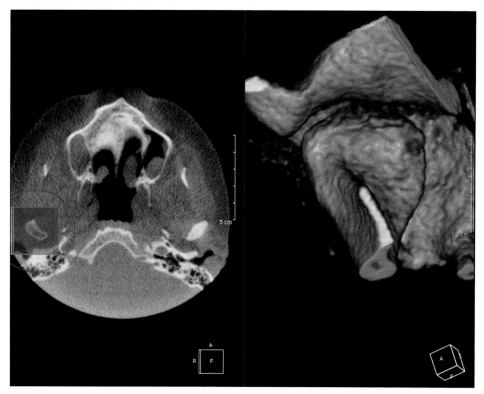

Fig 12-1c The right condyle is reconstructed by using the Cube tool. Note the inflammatory changes in the antra.

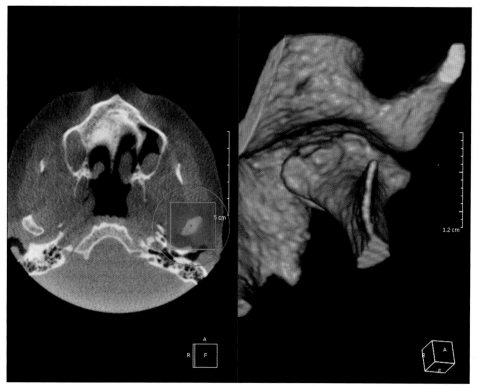

Fig 12-1d The left condyle is reconstructed by using the Cube tool. Compare this condyle to the right-side image in Fig 12-1c.

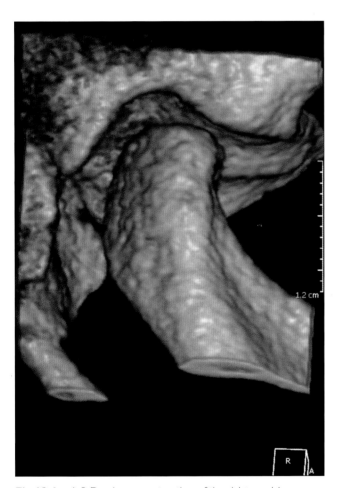

Fig 12-1e A 3-D color reconstruction of the right condyle.

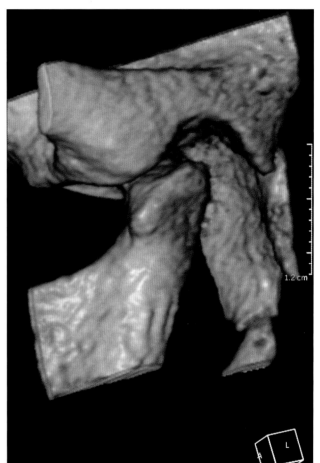

Fig 12-1f Note the difference between Fig 12-1e and this 3-D color reconstruction of the left condyle.

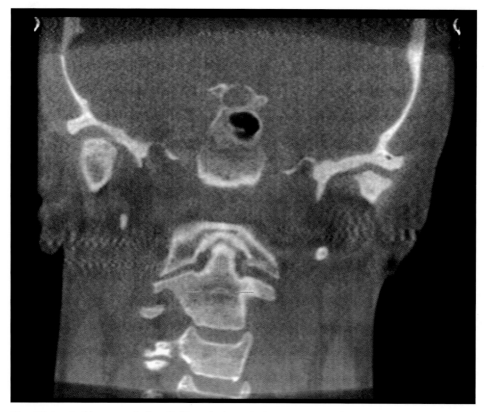

Fig 12-1g A thin coronal slice (0.15 mm) through the midregion of the condyles demonstrates asymmetry.

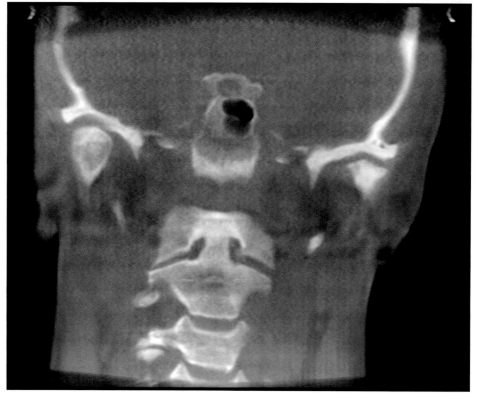

Fig 12-1h Same view as Fig 12-1g, presented in a 20.0-mm slice.

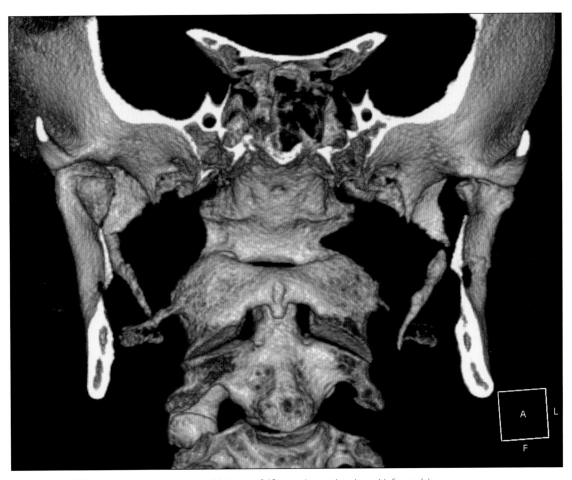

Fig 12-1i A 3-D color reconstruction at a thickness of 40 mm shows the altered left condyle.

FIG
12-2

FACIAL ASYMMETRY

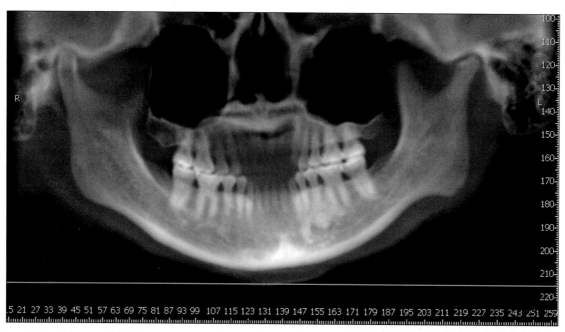

Fig 12-2a A 33-year-old white woman was referred to a Seattle, Washington, imaging center for evaluation of a facial asymmetry. A panoramic reconstruction shows left-side hypoplasia. The teeth are in occlusion. Note the presence of mandibular tori.

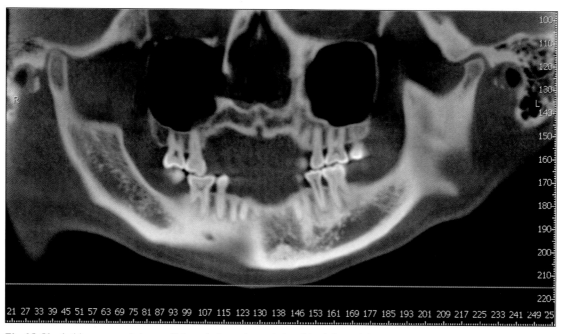

Fig 12-2b A thin panoramic image (2.0 mm) shows hypoplasia of the left condylar neck and head.

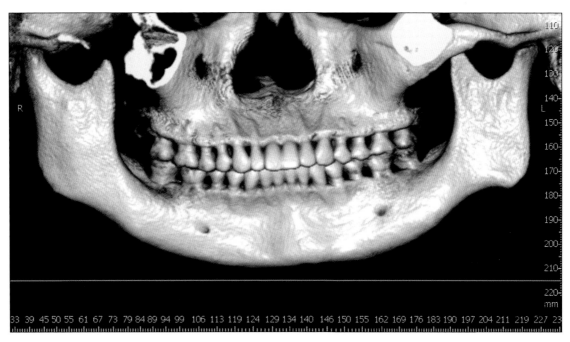

Fig 12-2c A 3-D color panoramic reconstruction shows hypoplasia of the left condylar neck and head, and the teeth are in occlusion. The midlines are aligned.

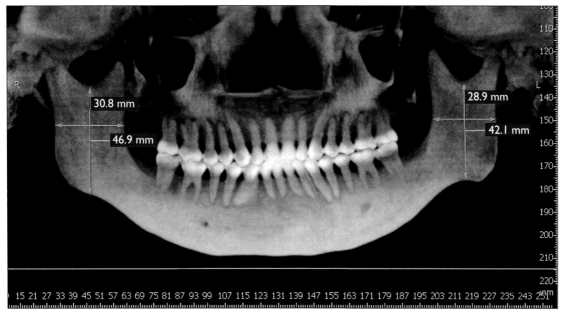

Fig 12-2d A maximum intensity projection image with measurements reveals that the entire ramus is hypoplastic. This finding, coupled with the hypoplastic neck and condylar head, confirms hypoplasia of the entire left ramus.

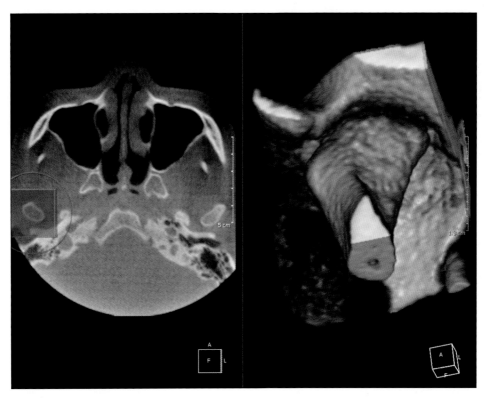

Fig 12-2e The right condylar head in a 3-D color reconstruction.

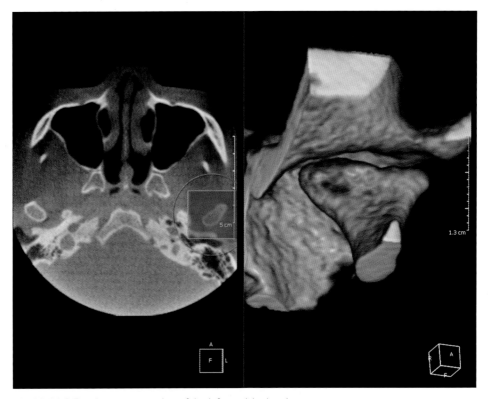

Fig 12-2f 3-D color reconstruction of the left condylar head.

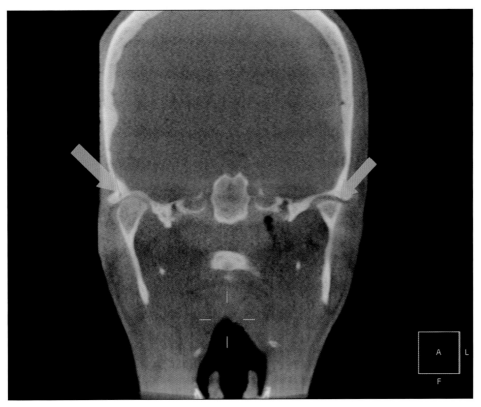

Fig 12-2g A coronal slice demonstrates the hypoplastic left condyle in comparison with the right condyle (*arrows*).

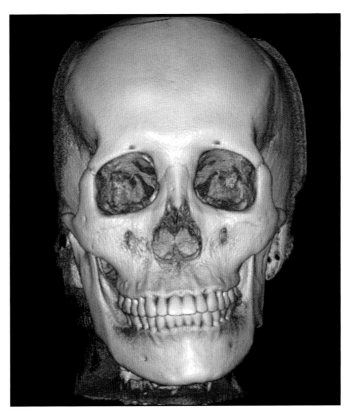

Fig 12-2h A 3-D color reconstruction of the skull shows the shortened left side. Note the difference between the left and right mandibular angles.

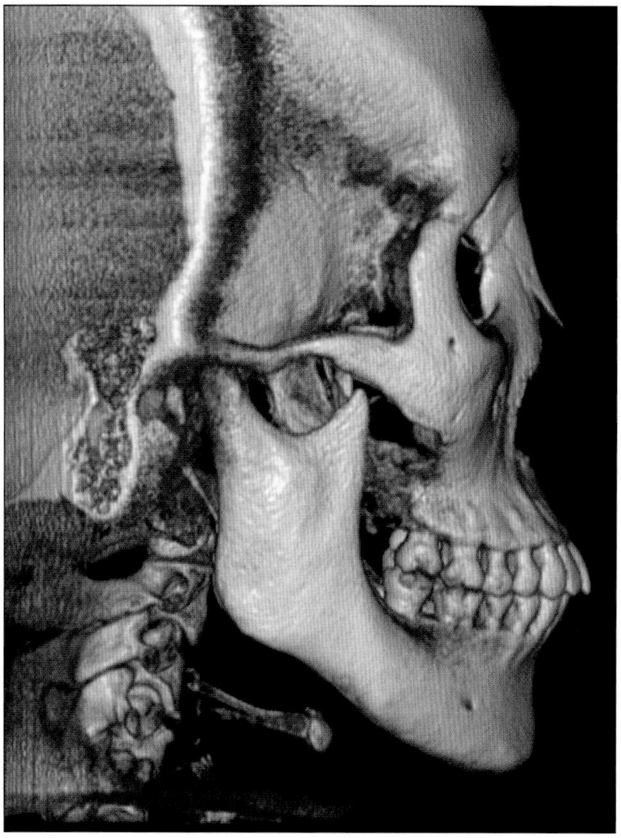

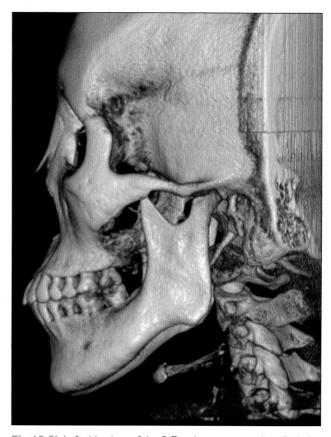

Fig 12-2i Right-side view of the 3-D color reconstruction.

Fig 12-2j Left-side view of the 3-D color reconstruction displaying smaller structures than those in Fig 12-2i.

Fig

12-3

BILATERAL CONDYLAR REMODELING

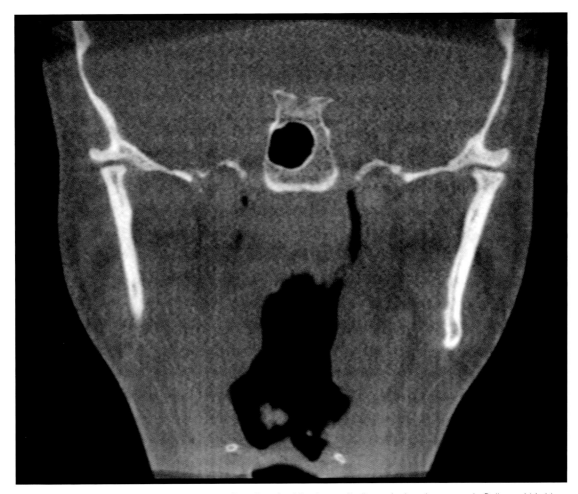

Fig 12-3a A 31-year-old white woman was referred to the Northwest Radiography imaging center in Bellevue, Washington, for evaluation of the TMJs. The symmetric changes suggest an autoimmune problem such as rheumatoid arthritis. This thin coronal slice shows bilateral remodeling and flattening of the condylar heads.

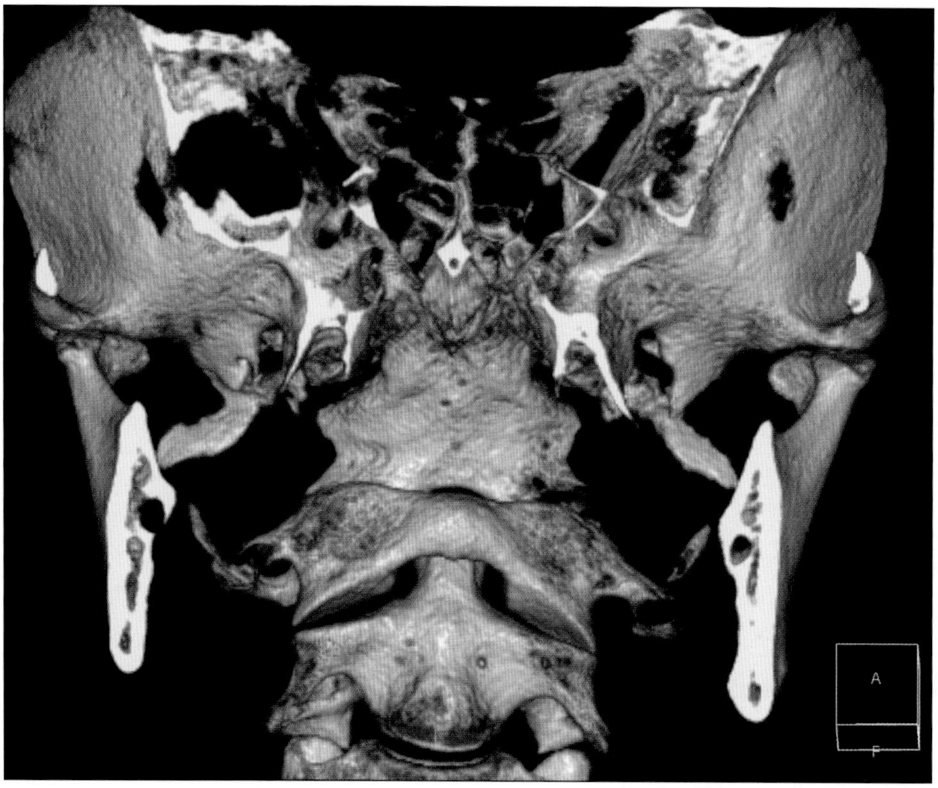

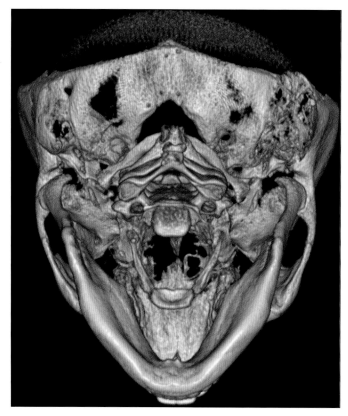

Fig 12-3b This 3-D color reconstruction confirms the bilateral remodeling and flattening of the condylar heads seen in Fig 12-3a.

Fig 12-3c A 3-D color reconstruction viewed from the foot end reveals a rather symmetric relationship of the condyles and fossae.

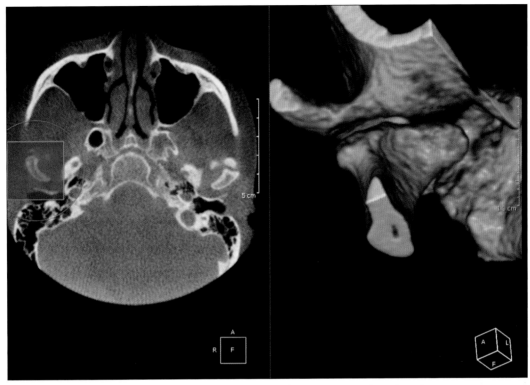

Fig 12-3d The Cube tool is used to show the right condyle in an anteroposterior orientation.

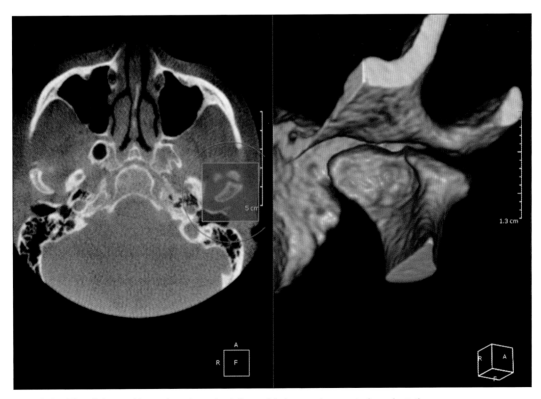

Fig 12-3e The Cube tool is used to show the left condyle in an anteroposterior orientation.

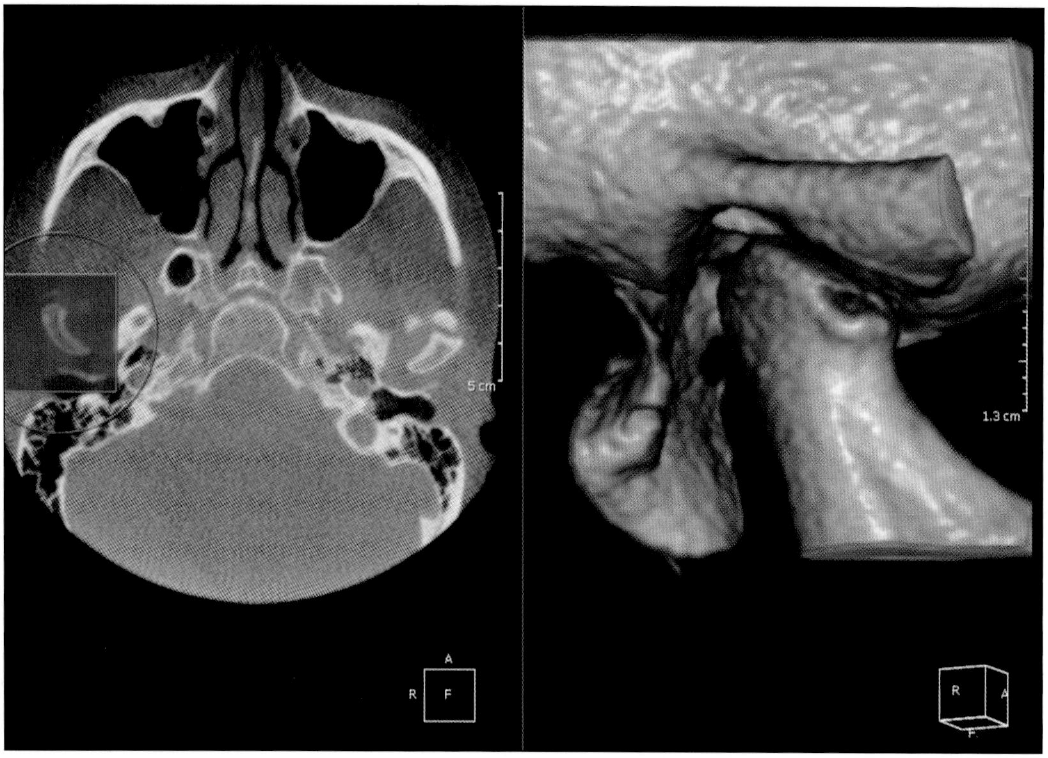

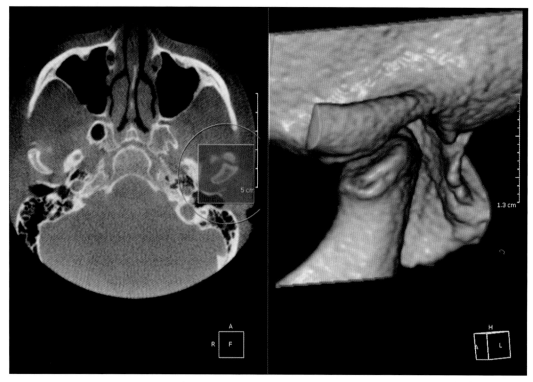

Fig 12-3f The Cube tool is used to show the right condyle in a lateral orientation.

Fig 12-3g The Cube tool is used to show the left condyle in a lateral orientation.

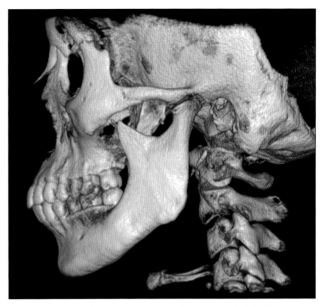

Fig 12-3h 3-D color reconstruction of the patient's right side.

Fig 12-3i 3-D color reconstruction of the patient's left side.

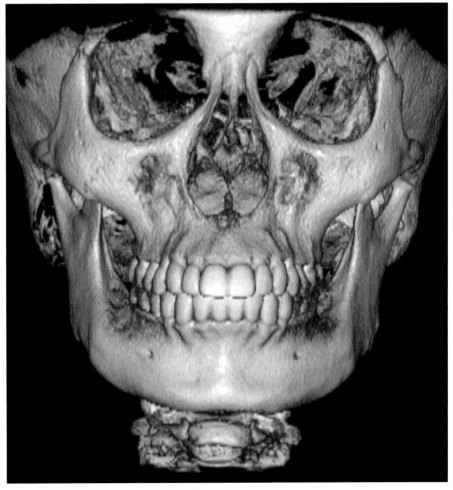

Fig 12-3j A 3-D color reconstruction of the patient from an anterior view shows the obvious mandibular symmetry despite the gross condylar changes.

FIG

12-4

OSTEOARTHRITIS OF THE TMJ STRUCTURES

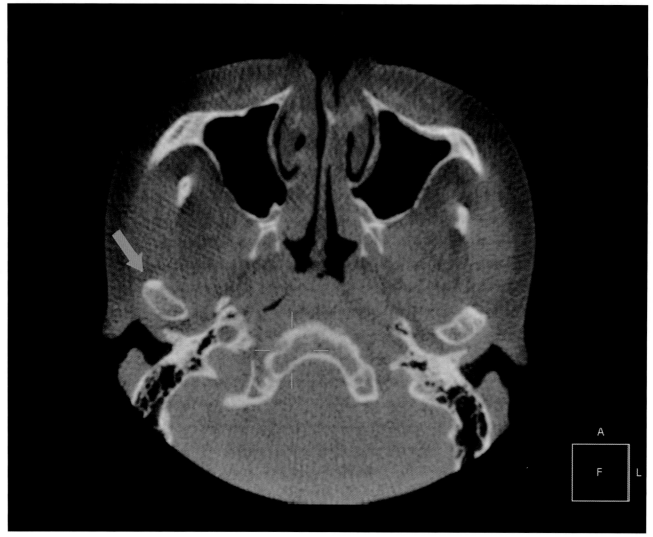

Fig 12-4a This case represents a 34-year-old white woman with mild, intermittent, unilateral joint pain. In the past, the term *bird beak* was frequently applied to changes associated with osteoarthritis (OA) of the TMJ, probably because of the myriad lateral projection techniques applied to see the condylar change. Now that it is possible to visualize the condylar structures in 3-D color reconstructions, some of the terminology should be reconsidered. A thin axial slice (0.15 mm) of the midregion of the condyles reveals some condylar sclerosis on the lateral pole of the right condyle *(arrow)*.

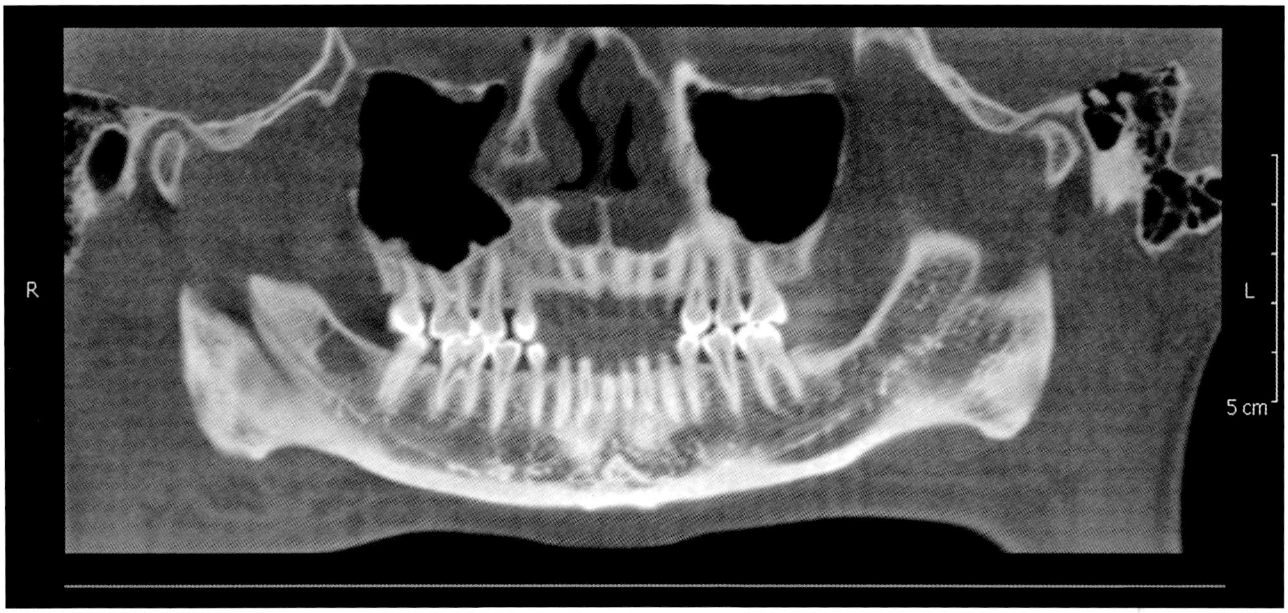

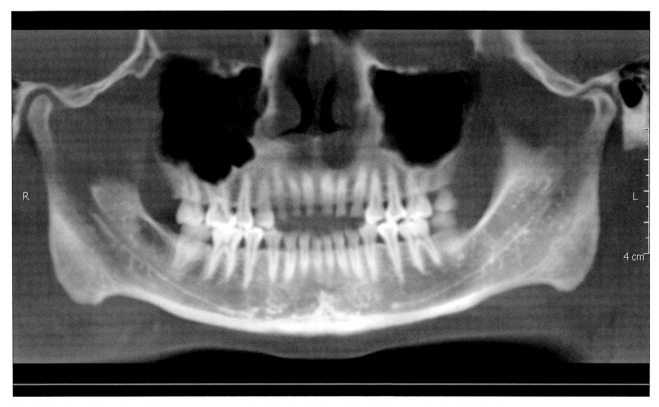

Fig 12-4b In this thin slice pseudopanoramic reconstruction, the left condyle shows what appears to be an osteophytic projection, or what some have called a classic *bird-beak* appearance.

Fig 12-4c In a thicker slice of the panoramic reconstruction, the left condyle still demonstrates the bird-beak appearance.

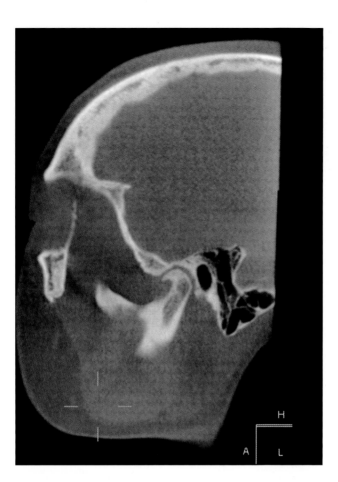

Fig 12-4d Even this thin slice sagittal view suggests the same appearance as in Fig 12-4c.

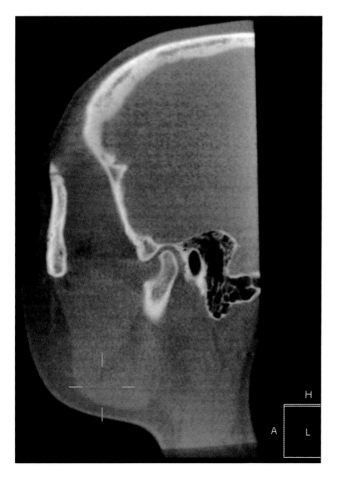

Fig 12-4e The condyle on the patient's right side appears to be normal in this saggital view.

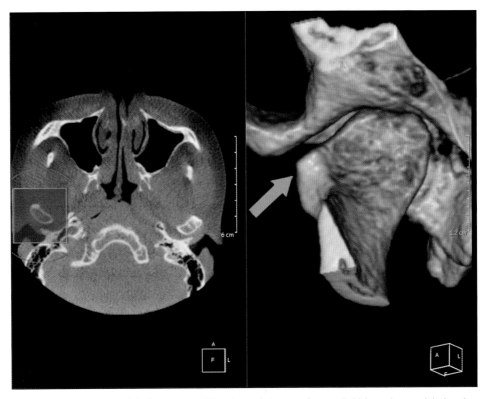

Fig 12-4f The right condyle is *not* normal, but instead shows a flattened, thickened, remodeled region *(arrow)* on the lateral pole as suggested in the axial image, Fig 12-4a.

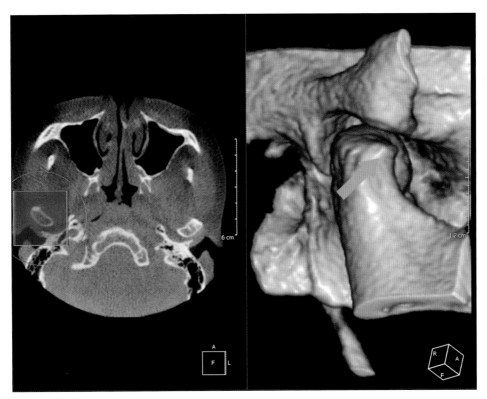

Fig 12-4g The right condyle seen from the lateral view confirms a flattened, thickened, remodeled area *(arrow)*; one might imagine that in a 2-D lateral grayscale image, this region would look like a beak.

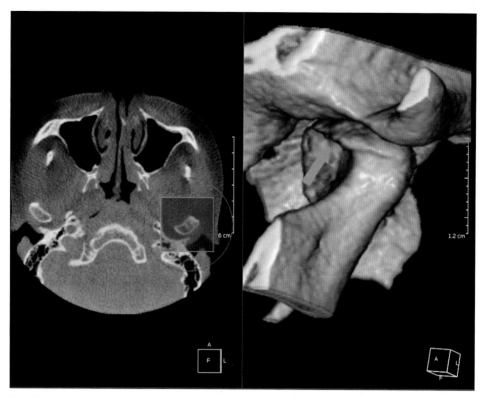

Fig 12-4h The view of the left condyle in 3-D color with the use of the Cube tool reveals some significant lipping of the bone along the anterior margin *(arrow)*. Compare this image to Fig 12-4i to see how the bird-beak appearance could also have been misinterpreted by simple angulation changes.

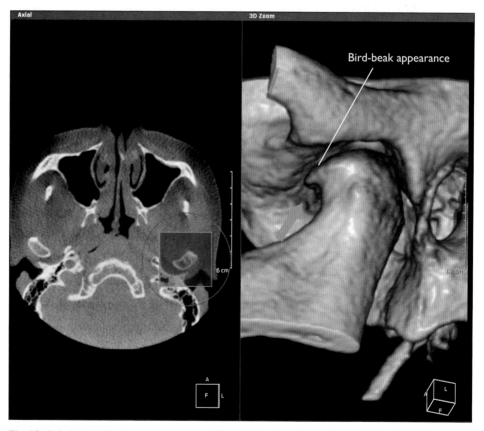

Fig 12-4i Is it a bird-beak appearance or not? You decide after comparison with Fig 12-4h.

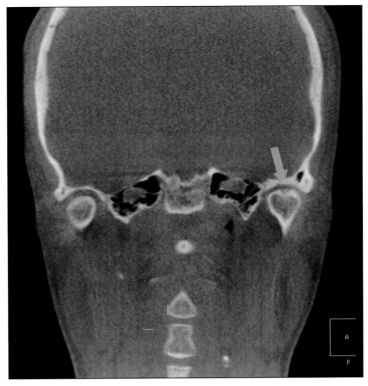

Fig 12-4j This coronal slice shows a subchondral cyst on the superior aspect of the left condyle *(arrow)*.

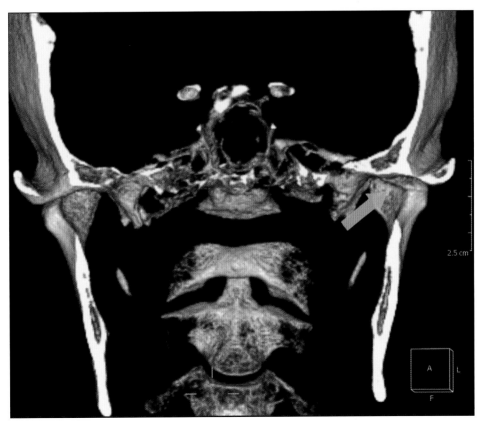

Fig 12-4k A 3-D color reconstruction illustrates the lipping phenomenon *(arrow)*, but does not show the cyst seen in Fig 12-4j. As detailed as CBVI views can be, multiple images from the data volume are usually required to visualize all of the changes and problems.

FIG
12-5

LOOSE BODY IN THE JOINT SPACE

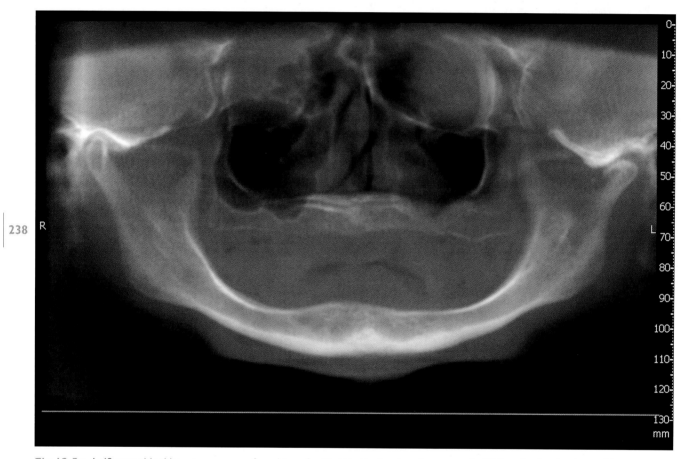

238   R   L

Fig 12-5a A 62-year-old white woman was referred to a Seattle, Washington, imaging center for TMJ evaluation because of joint noises. A panoramic reconstruction from the data volume shows little indication of a loose body in the joint space (also known as a *joint mouse*), although the left condylar head is altered in appearance.

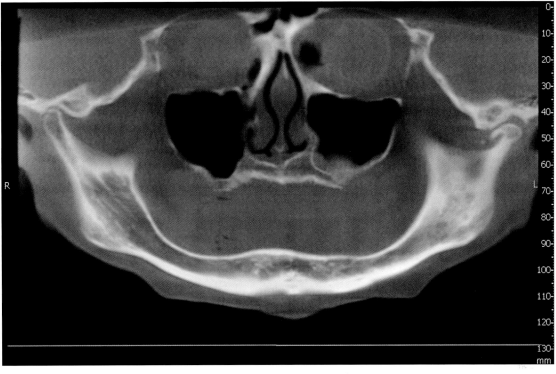

Fig 12-5b A thin slice pseudopanoramic reconstruction shows a very slight radiopacity anterior to the left condylar head.

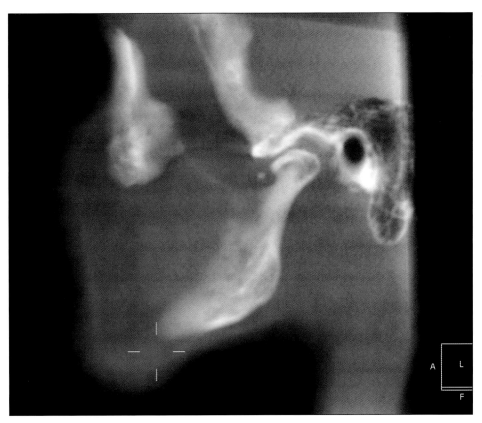

Fig 12-5c A sagittal slice at a thickness of approximately 20 mm simulates the typical plain image view one might see in tomography. The loose body is clearly depicted.

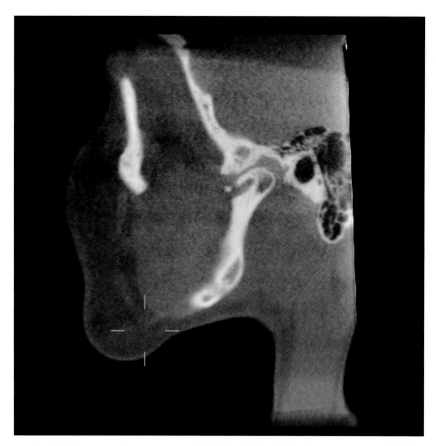

Fig 12-5d A thin sagittal slice (0.15 mm) demonstrates the loose body more precisely.

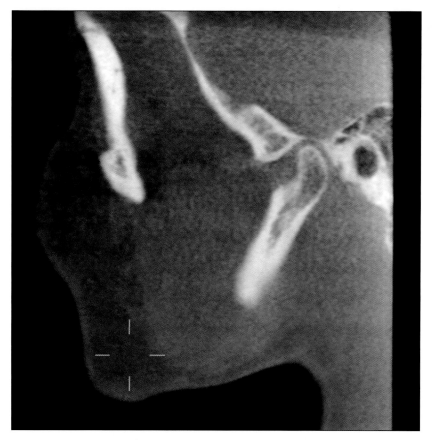

Fig 12-5e A thin sagittal slice (0.15 mm) of the normal right side is provided for comparison.

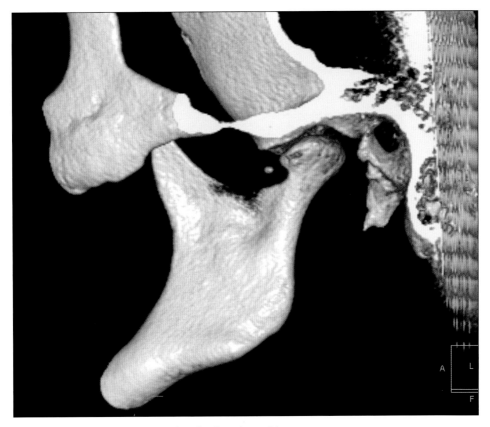

Fig 12-5f A 3-D color reconstruction visualizes the problem.

241

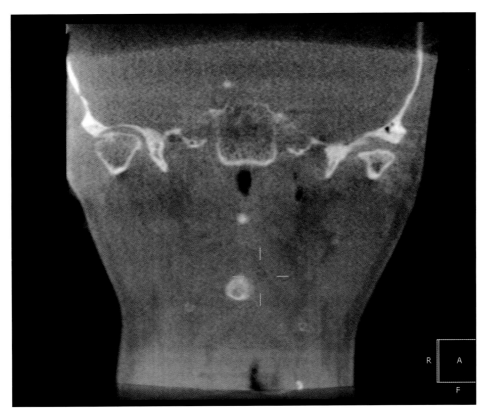

Fig 12-5g A coronal view is used to compare the left and right sides. The left condyle is hypoplastic and shows an altered morphology. The right condyle has some less dramatic changes.

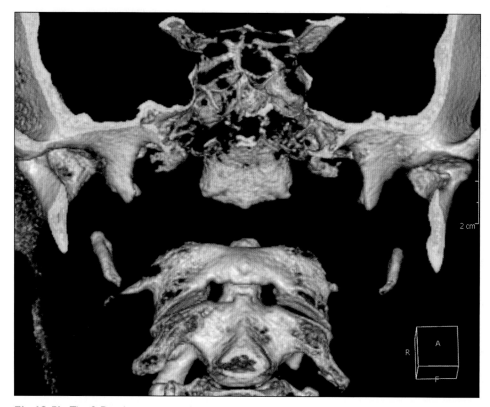

Fig 12-5h The 3-D color reconstruction compares left and right sides. The left condyle is hypoplastic; lipping is evident. The loose body is not very apparent.

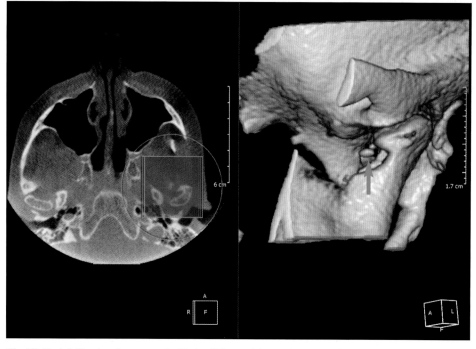

Fig 12-5i A 3-D color view created with the Cube tool shows the loose body in the left condyle *(arrow)*.

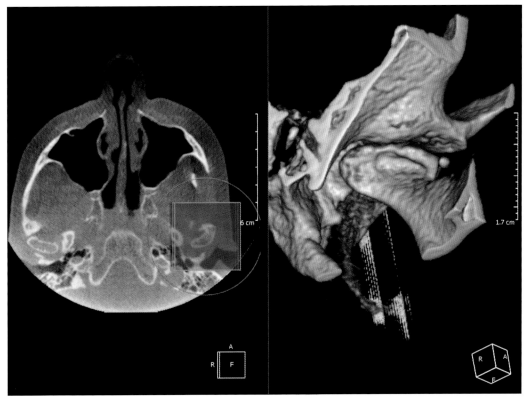

Fig 12-5j A 3-D color view created with the Cube tool shows the left condyle in an anterior projection, revealing the loose body adjacent to the lateral pole.

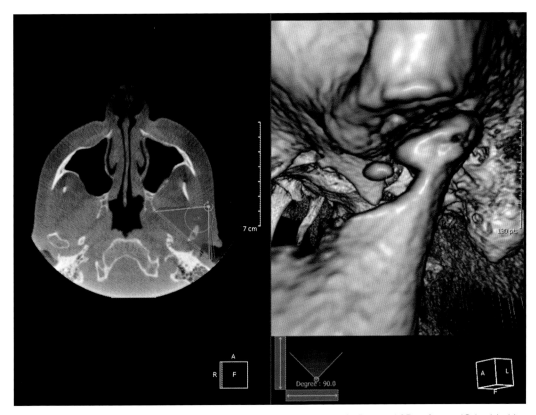

Fig 12-5k The left condyle is shown in 3-D color Endoscope mode in OnDemand 3D software (CyberMed International). Note how this tool increases the image resolution significantly.

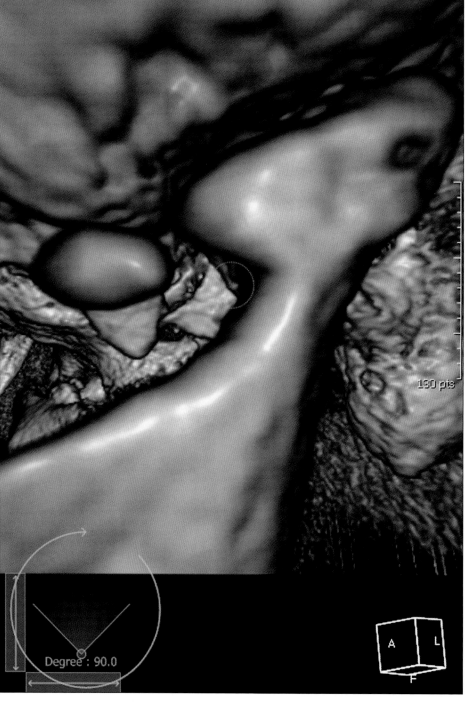

Fig 12-51 Enlargement of the Endoscope view.

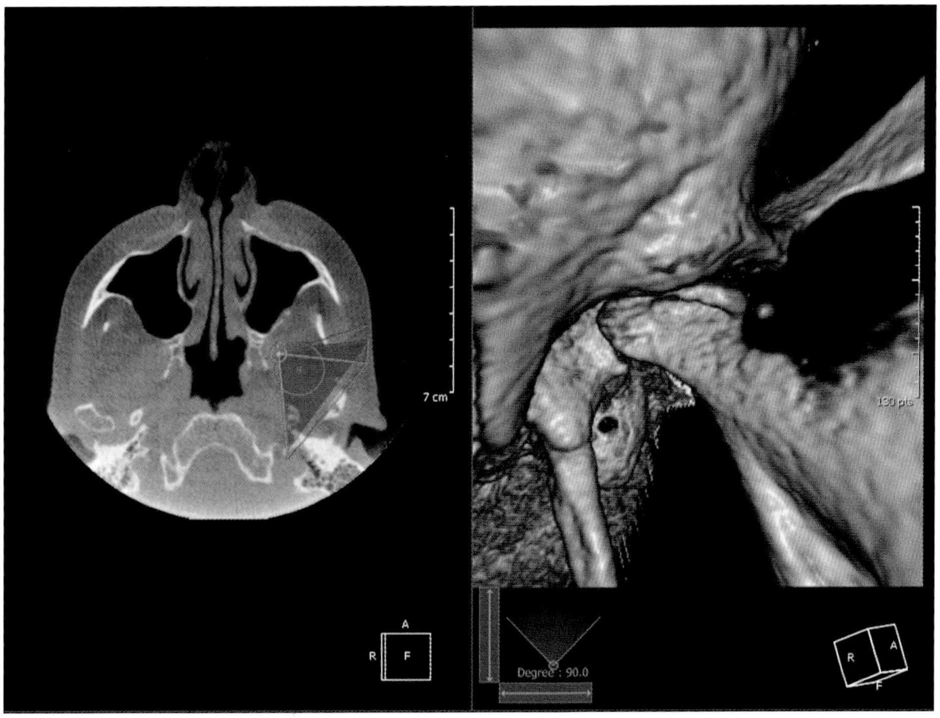

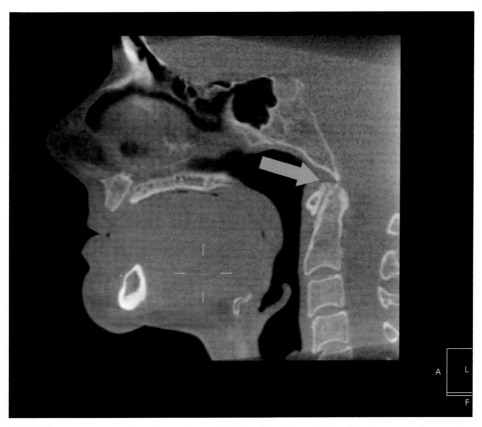

Fig 12-5m An Endoscope view from the anterior perspective shows the condyle at a distance.

Fig 12-5n A thin sagittal slice shows the vertebral bodies. Osteophytic activity is seen on the superior portion of C2 *(arrow)*. Changes in the vertebral bodies are often seen concomitantly with condylar changes from OA.

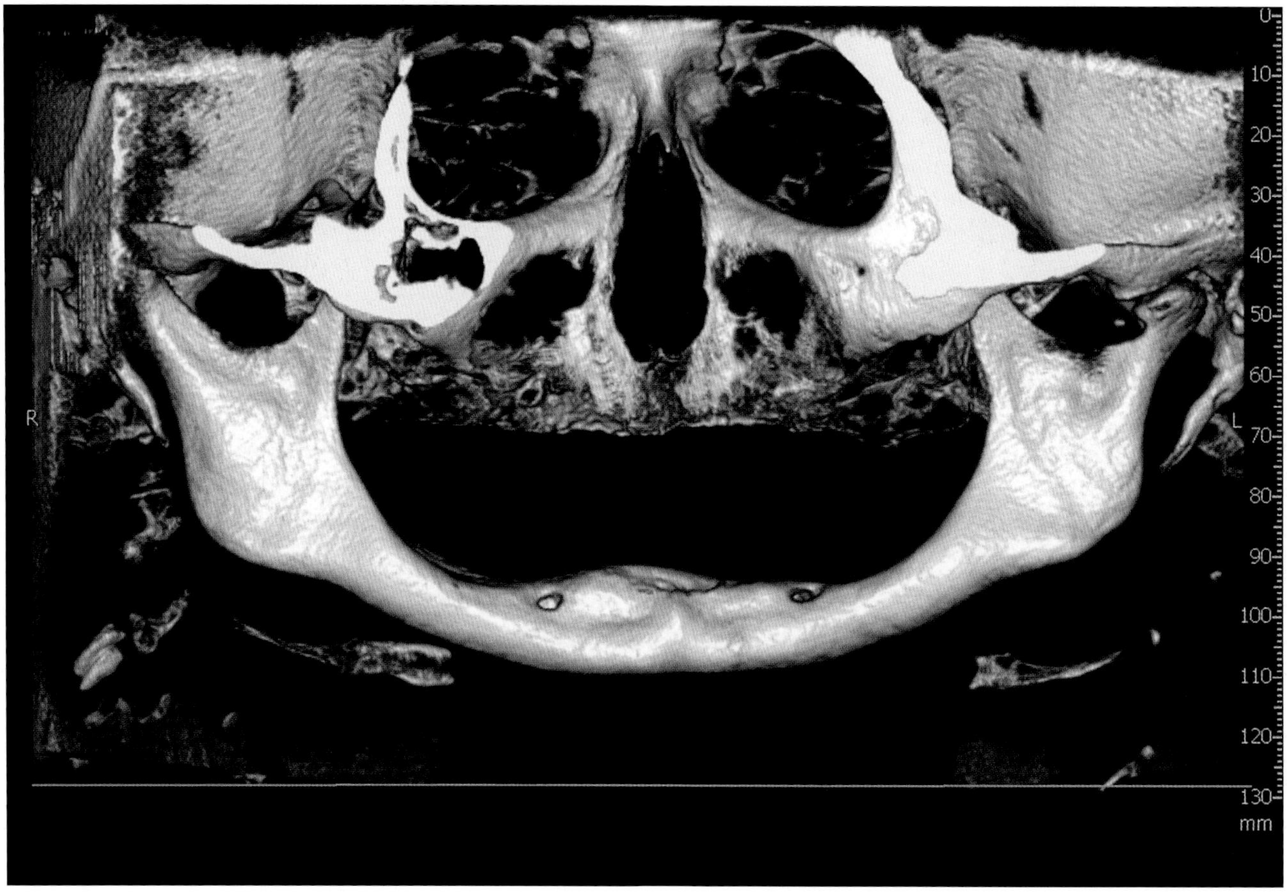

Fig 12-5o A 3-D color panoramic reconstruction demonstrates the condylar changes, including the hypoplastic left condylar neck and head.

FIG
12-6

CONDYLAR TUMOR

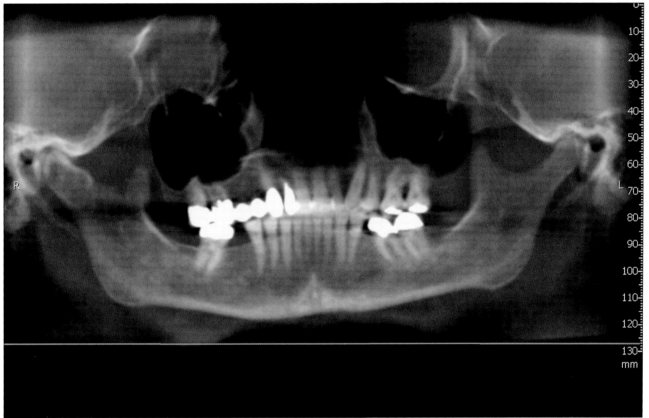

Fig 12-6a A 62-year-old white woman was referred to Advanced Dental Imaging in Salem, New Hampshire, for evaluation of a proposed implant site for a missing maxillary right lateral incisor, as well as for evaluation of the TMJs. A panoramic reconstruction demonstrates an enlargement of the right condylar neck and head relative to the left side. The right stylohyoid process also appears elongated compared to the left.

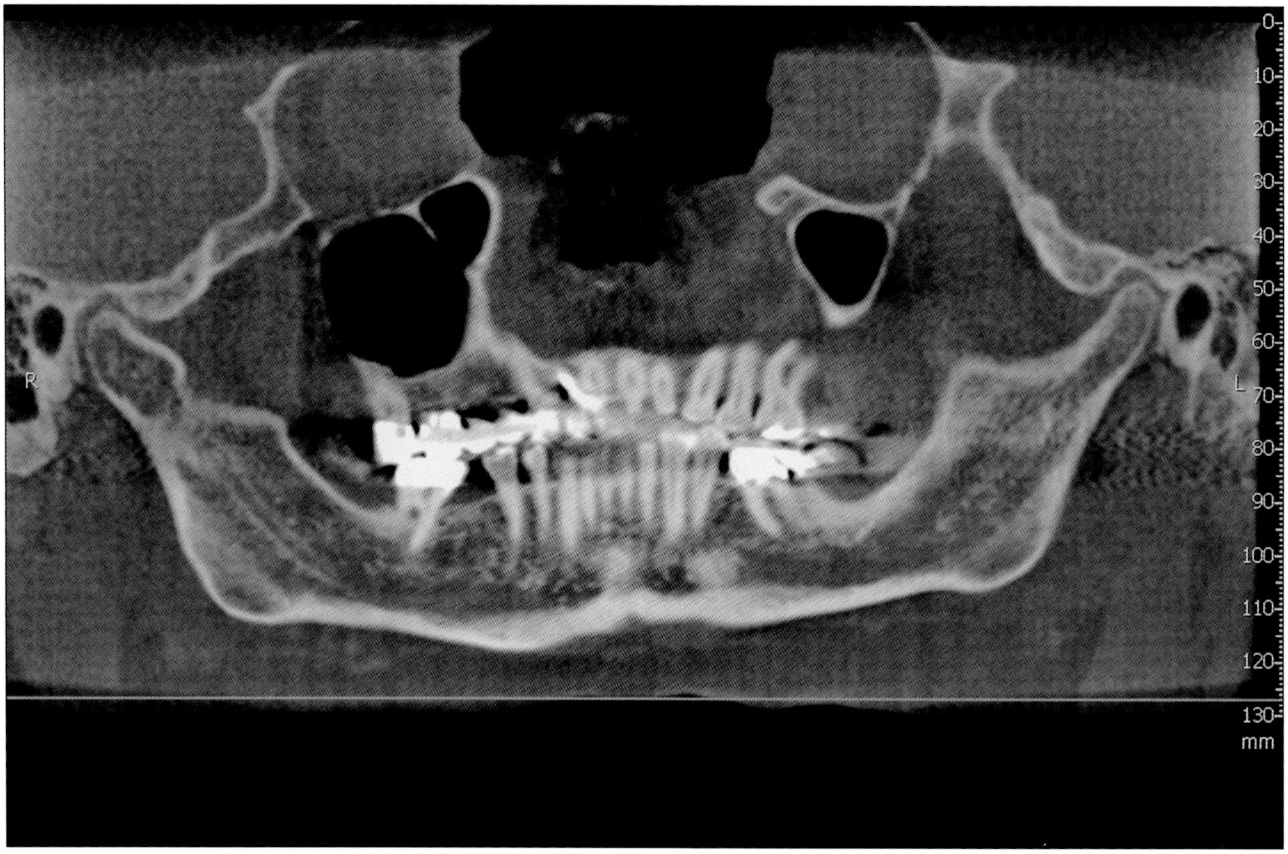

248

Fig 12-6b A thin slice (0.15 mm) pseudopanoramic reconstruction confirms the altered right condylar morphology and enlarged size.

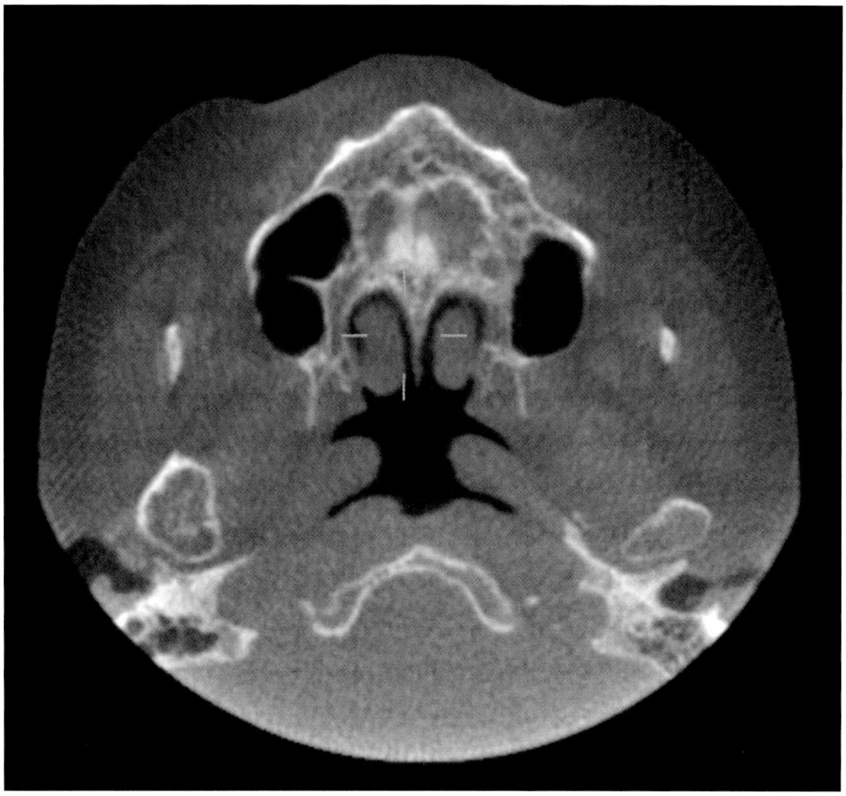

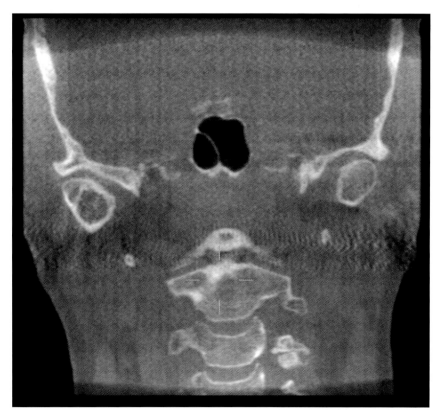

Fig 12-6c A thin axial slice (0.15 mm) allows the clinician to compare the right and left condylar heads.

249

Fig 12-6d A thin coronal slice (0.15 mm) allows the clinician to compare the right and left condylar heads. Note the appearance of two loculi on the right condyle.

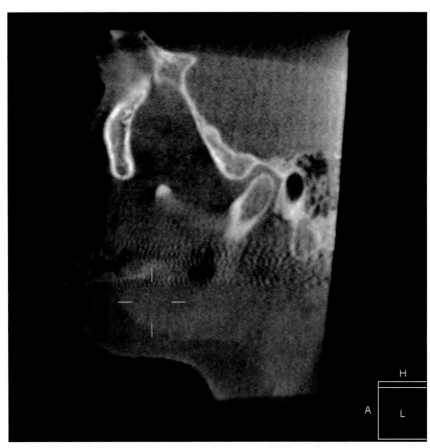

Fig 12-6e A thin sagittal slice (0.15 mm) shows the normal left condyle.

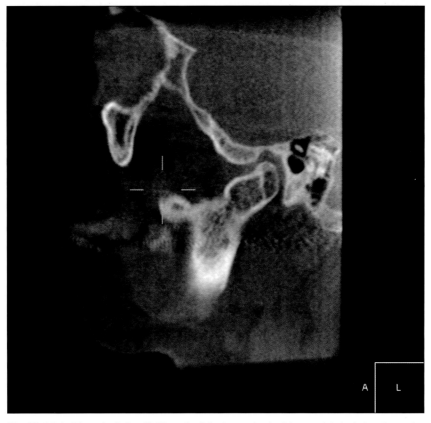

Fig 12-6f A thin sagittal slice (0.15 mm) of the hyperplastic right condyle includes the neck.

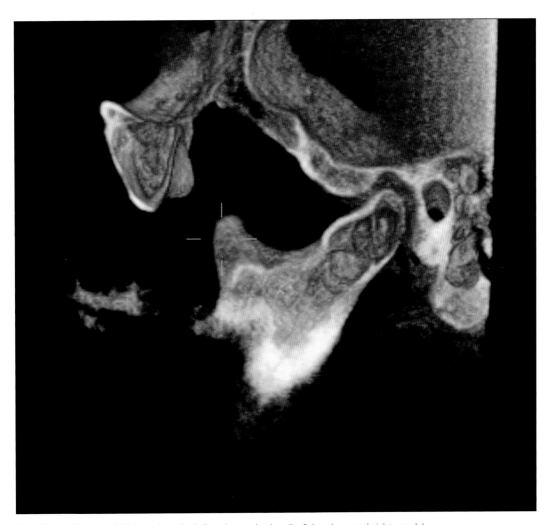

Fig 12-6g A thicker (10.1 mm) sagittal slice shows the loculi of the abnormal right condyle.

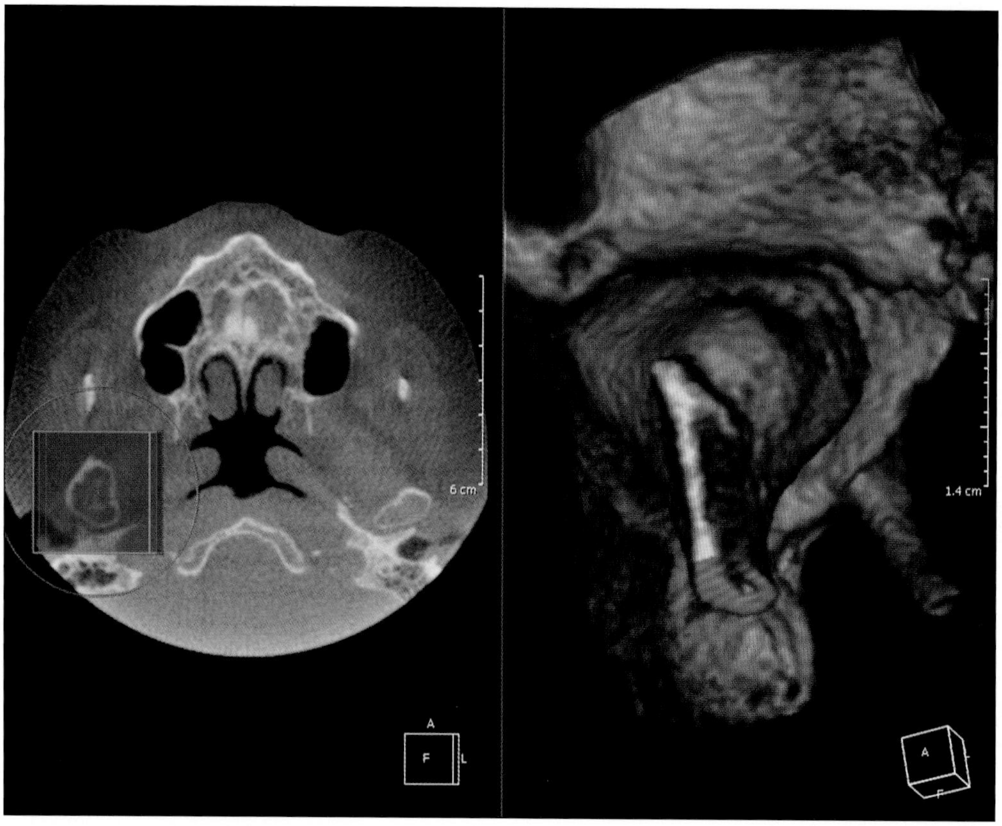

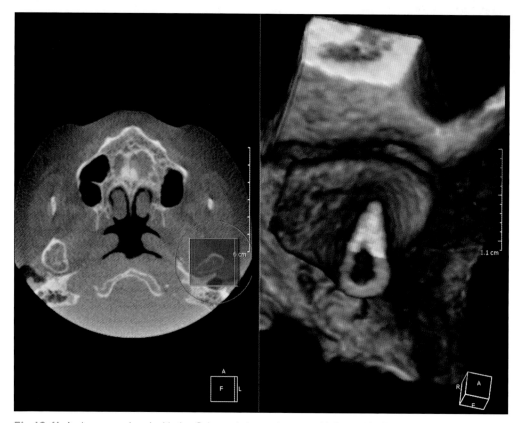

Fig 12-6h An image rendered with the Cube tool shows the enlarged condyle. The tumor is apparently originating from the pterygoid fovea region.

Fig 12-6i An image rendered with the Cube tool shows the normal left condyle for comparison.

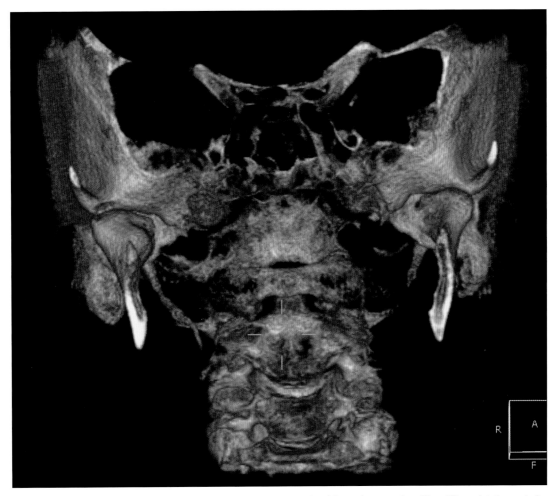

Fig 12-6j A 3-D color reconstruction shows the TMJ structures in a bilateral comparison. The differential diagnosis for this lesion included central giant cell granuloma, hyperplasia of the right condyle, osteochondroma, and traumatic bone cyst.

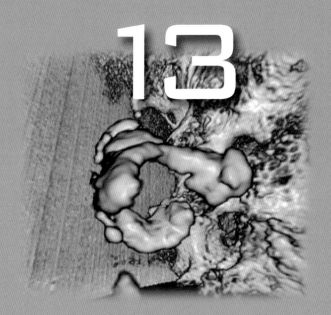

13

SYSTEMIC FINDINGS

Although patients who visit our dental practices can have many different systemic conditions (eg, cardiopulmonary problems, endocrine disorders, and so on), few of them will show overt radiographic signs of their disorders in the head and neck region when imaged. Recent clinical studies have identified the presence of sclerotic plaques in the carotid region as a potential harbinger of hypertension and possibly stroke,[1–3] and there are always patients who are referred to imaging centers if various head or neck cancers are suspected. Regardless, significant systemic findings are rare in the typical population of patients that we treat and refer for cone beam volumetric imaging (CBVI). This is the good news.

The bad news, however, is that although the incidence of occult pathology may be small, the outcome could be significant for the patient with a positive finding. *I must reiterate here the absolute requirement for the entire data volume to be examined by a competent radiologist, with either a medical or oral and maxillofacial background, if we are to properly use CBVI for* our patients' needs. A myopic clinician may become involved in a serious lawsuit if no attempt is made to examine the data volume beyond an implant site assessment or evaluation for a clicking joint. These CBVI data volumes are not the single radiographs used in the past for most clinical decisions. The scans produce powerful, reconstructable data sets that require the clinician to have significant anatomic and pathologic understanding as well as the skills for thorough patient examination and precise radiographic interpretation.

The following cases demonstrate some of the serious systemic findings reported in more than 1,800 patients. There is no doubt that, as more cases are examined worldwide and the findings reported, many more significant systemic findings will be uncovered in these CBVI data volumes.

One systemic condition or disorder that appears to have identifiable radiographic findings in the CBVI data volumes in its later stages is type 2 diabetes mellitus. I have examined more than 1,000 data volumes to date, and I believe that I have seen medial arterial calcinosis (MAC), formerly called *Mönckeberg sclerosis*, in at least 13 cases. Although that translates into an incidence of only 1.3%, this finding is significant. Type 2 diabetes mellitus is predicted to affect over 200 million people worldwide by the year 2010.[4] The National Diabetes Education Program (NDEP), a branch of the US Department of Health and Human Services, only recently produced an informational brochure for dental clinicians to discuss with and give to patients. The NDEP states that "nearly 21 million Americans have diabetes, and some 7 million don't know they have it."[5]

MAC is a unique problem for diabetic patients. Vessels with calcifications in their medial layers cannot respond appropriately to the vascular demands placed on them. This is a form of peripheral arterial disease (PAD), which is significant because it could lead to below-the-knee amputations in diabetic patients with end-stage renal disease (ESRD). The NDEP reports that diabetes is responsible for "fully 67% of lower-extremity amputations."[5] In my experience, MAC can be seen on panoramic and even intraoral films.[6,7] We have known

about the problem for years, but now we have an incredible opportunity to visualize the changes in carotid arteries through CBVI. The following cases illustrate this convincingly. It is likely that some of the cases described in the literature as having "diffuse calcifications," suggesting a patient is at increased risk for stroke, may have grossly underestimated cases of type 2 diabetes mellitus; the panoramic image is a vastly inferior image modality for this type of evaluation. It also underscores the necessity for the radiologist or clinician to have all of the clinical information while examining CBVI data volumes, so the findings can be placed in their proper context.

Type 2 diabetes mellitus is more common in African American, Hispanic, American Indian, Asian American, and Pacific Islander populations than in other populations. It is also more common in older members of the population.[5]

A quote from a recent article by researchers at the Cleveland Clinic Center for Continuing Education expertly sums up the relationship between type 2 diabetes mellitus and kidney function. These researchers state[8]:

Diabetes has become the number one cause of ESRD in the United States, and the incidence of type 2 diabetes mellitus continues to grow both in the United States and worldwide. Approximately 45% of new patients entering dialysis in the United States are diabetics. Early diagnosis of diabetes and early intervention are critical in preventing the normal progression to renal failure seen in many type 1 and a significant percentage of type 2 diabetics.

Diabetes is the number one cause of adult blindness and the number one cause of kidney failure. Two of every three people with diabetes die of heart disease or stroke.[5] Once thought of as an incidental finding, MAC is now considered to be a significant sign of PAD, which requires aggressive treatment in the diabetic patient.[9]

FIG

13-1

MEDIAL ARTERIAL CALCINOSIS: CASE 1

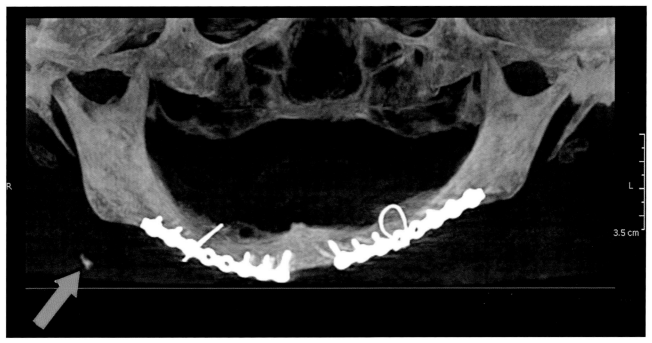

Fig 13-1a A 71-year-old white woman was referred to a Seattle, Washington, imaging service for follow-up evaluation of her mandibular surgery. A maximum intensity projection (MIP) panoramic image reveals a calcification in the right oropharyngeal area *(arrow)*. This projection appears very similar to calcifications seen in reports by Friedlander et al[1,2] and Carter et al.[3]

257

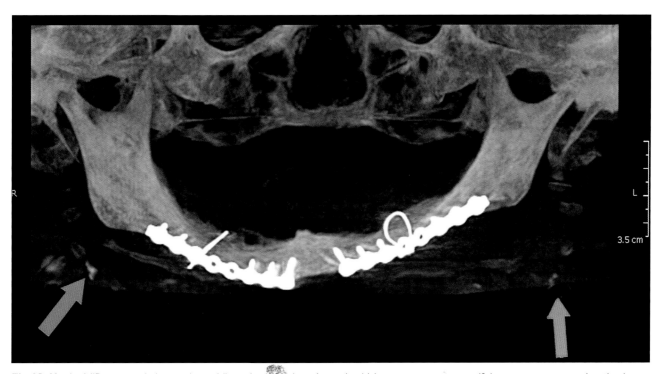

Fig 13-1b An MIP panoramic image shows bilateral calcifications *(arrows)*, which are very uncommon if the case represents sclerotic plaque. This presentation would be more consistent with a systemic condition that affects more of the vascular system, such as type 2 diabetes mellitus.

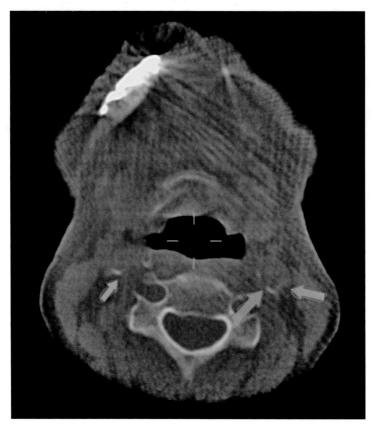

Fig 13-1c The axial view of this patient shows that the calcifications are starting to surround the carotid arteries (arrows).

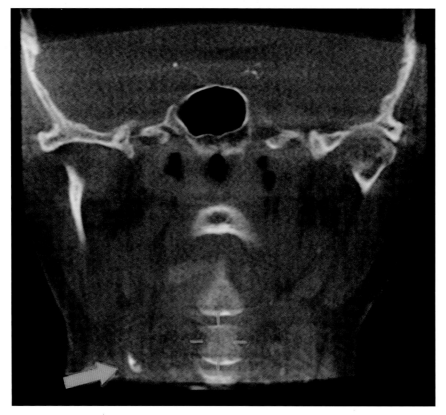

Fig 13-1d The coronal view of this patient shows the right-side calcification (arrow).

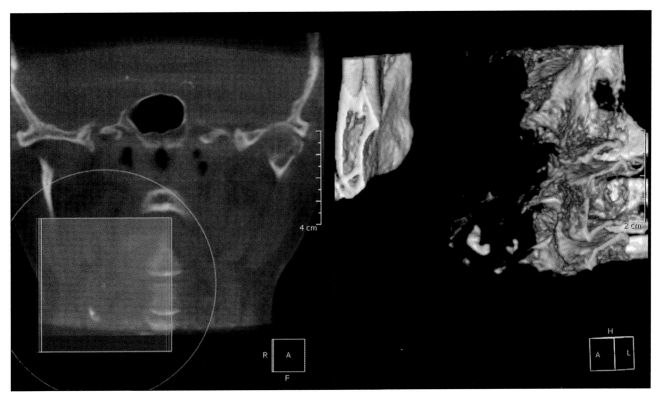

Fig 13-1e In the coronal section of the right-side calcification, the Cube tool reveals a more circumferential calcification pattern, like that seen in medial arterial calcinosis (MAC).

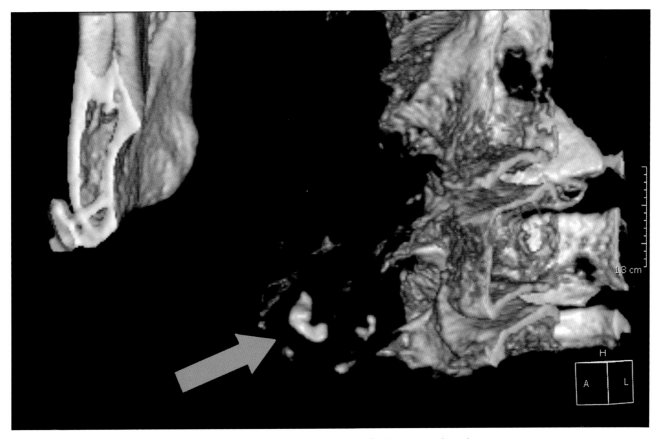

Fig 13-1f The image in Fig 13-1e is enlarged to reveal this circumferential calcification pattern *(arrow)*.

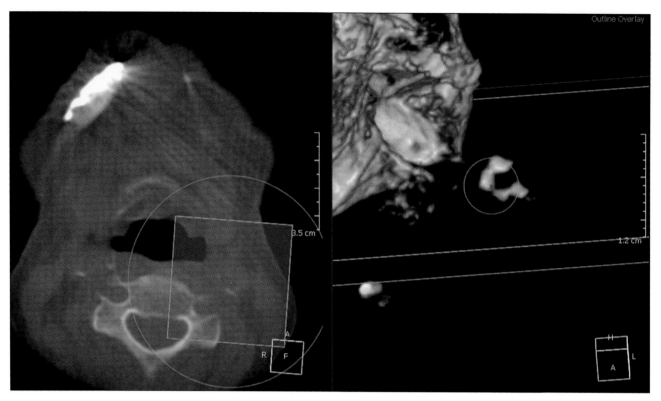

Fig 13-1g In the axial section of the left side, the Cube tool reveals the circumferential calcification pattern described previously.

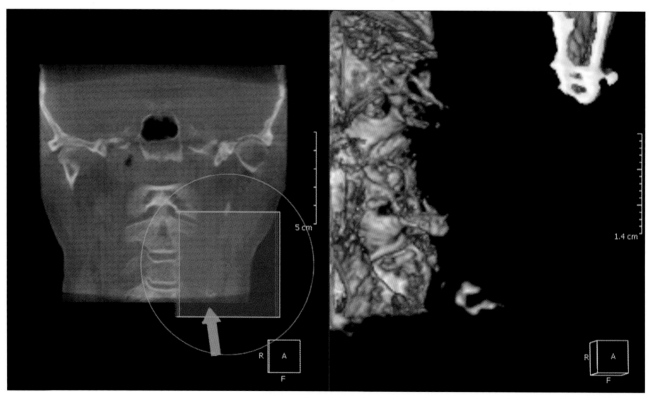

Fig 13-1h The Cube tool is used on the left side of the coronal section to help confirm the calcification *(arrow)*.

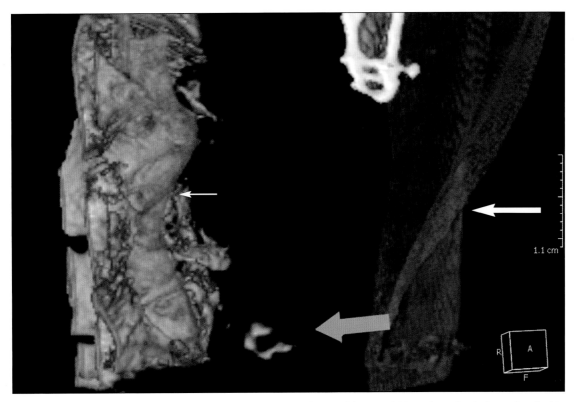

Fig 13-1i A 3-D color close-up of the left side confirms the calcification *(blue arrow)*. Note the patient's airway *(small white arrow)* and skin *(large white arrow)*.

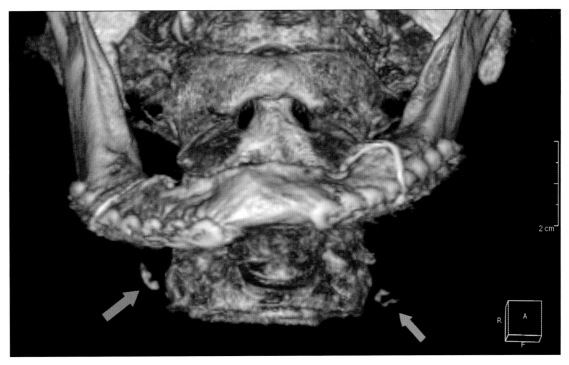

Fig 13-1j A 3-D color reconstruction shows both the result of orthognathic surgery and the bilateral MAC calcifications *(arrows)*.

FIG

13-2

MEDIAL ARTERIAL CALCINOSIS: CASE 2

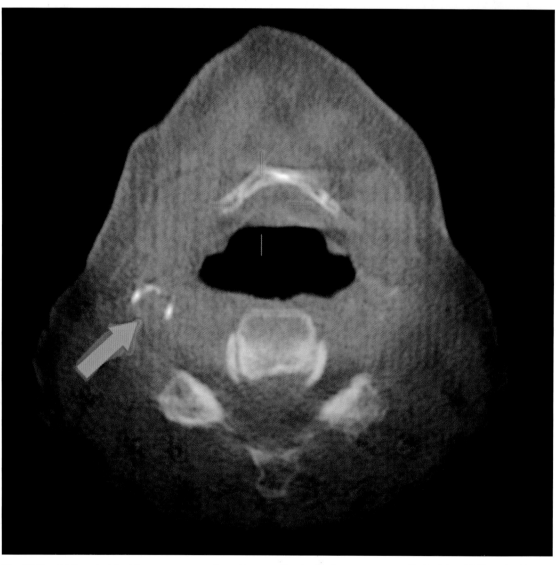

Fig 13-2a A 72-year-old white woman was referred to an orthodontist for temporomandibular joint (TMJ) evaluation related to moderate, intermittent joint pain. Type 2 diabetes mellitus is possibly the underlying systemic problem. A circumferential calcification *(arrow)* of the right carotid artery region is seen in this thin axial slice (0.15 mm).

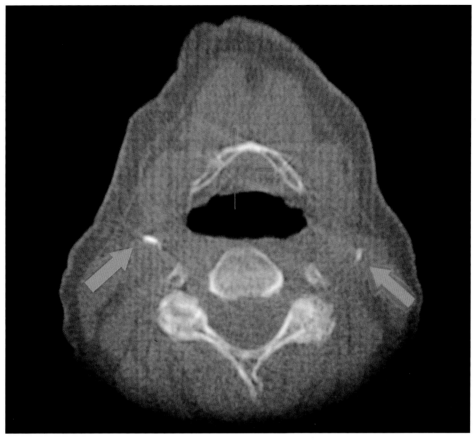

Fig 13-2b Bilateral calcifications *(arrows)* in the carotid artery regions are present at the level of C3 to C4.

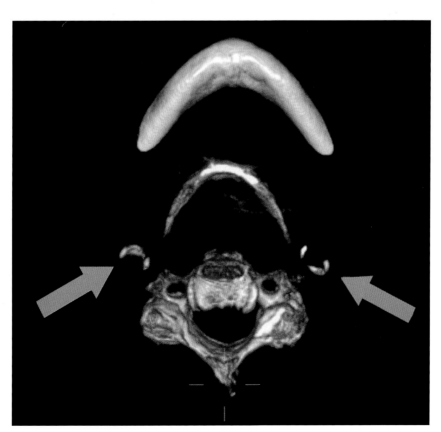

Fig 13-2c Bilateral circumferential calcifications *(arrows)* are confirmed in the 3-D color reconstruction.

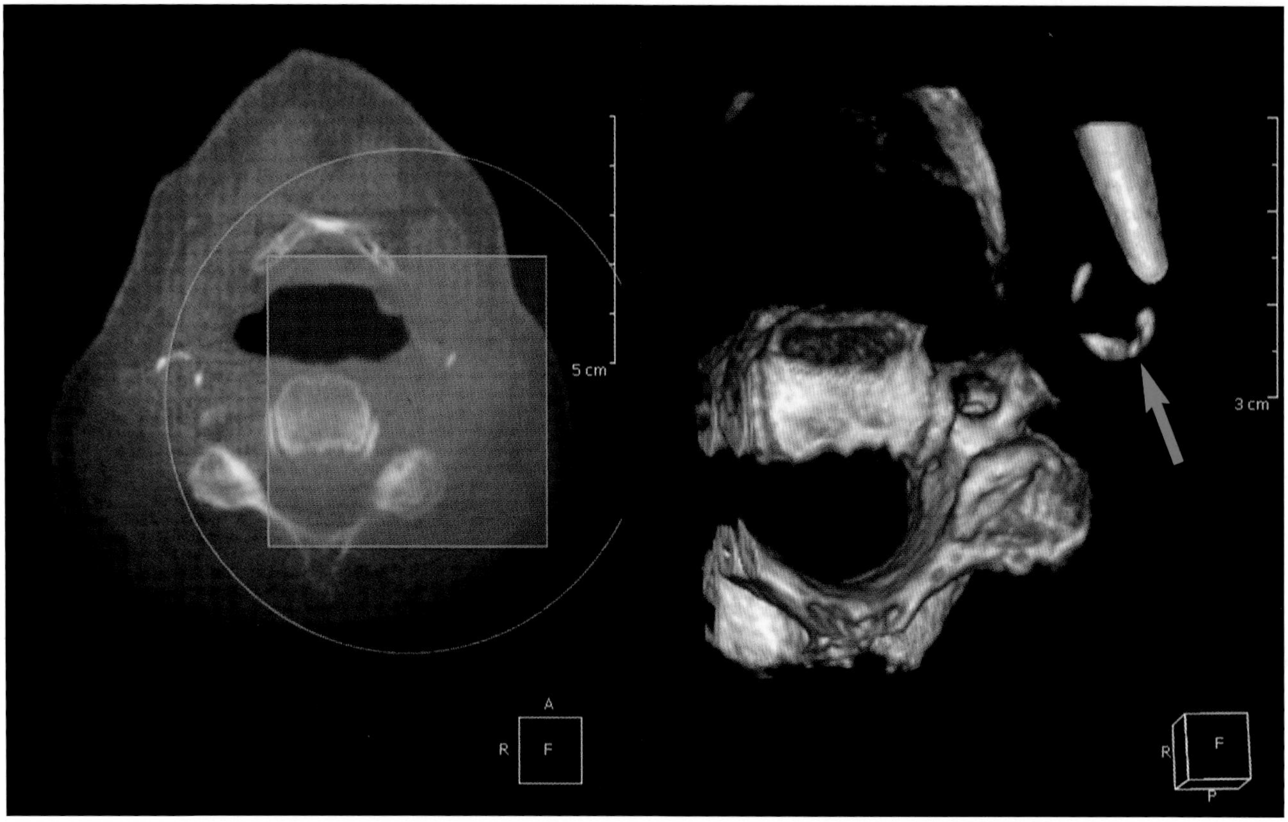

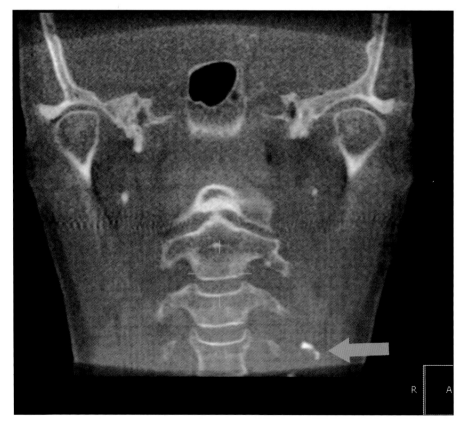

Fig 13-2d A Cube tool reconstruction of the left-side calcification *(arrow)* confirms the circumferential pattern.

Fig 13-2e Even this thin coronal slice (0.15 mm) suggests an MAC pattern *(arrow)*.

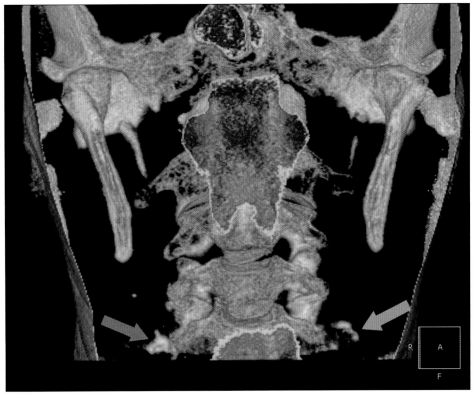

Fig 13-2f A 3-D color reconstruction shows bilateral calcifications *(arrows)*. Note the airway and condyle anatomy in this image. This was rendered at a thickness of about 40 mm.

265

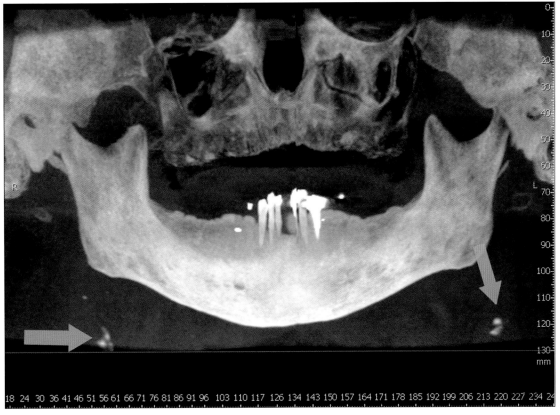

Fig 13-2g The MIP image also suggests the bilateral circumferential pattern of MAC *(arrows)*.

Fig

13-3

Medial Arterial Calcinosis: Case 3

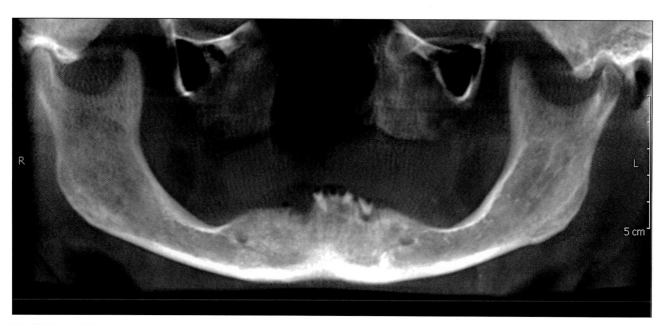

Fig 13-3a An 83-year-old white man was referred to the Northwest Radiography imaging center in Bellevue, Washington, for CBVI evaluation of implant sites. A panoramic reconstruction at a thickness of about 13 mm fails to show the oropharyngeal calcifications.

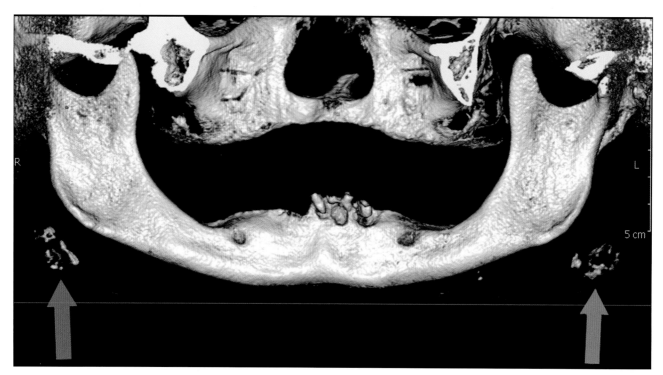

Fig 13-3b A 3-D color panoramic reconstruction at a thickness of about 30 mm clearly demonstrates the oropharyngeal calcifications consistent with MAC *(arrows)*.

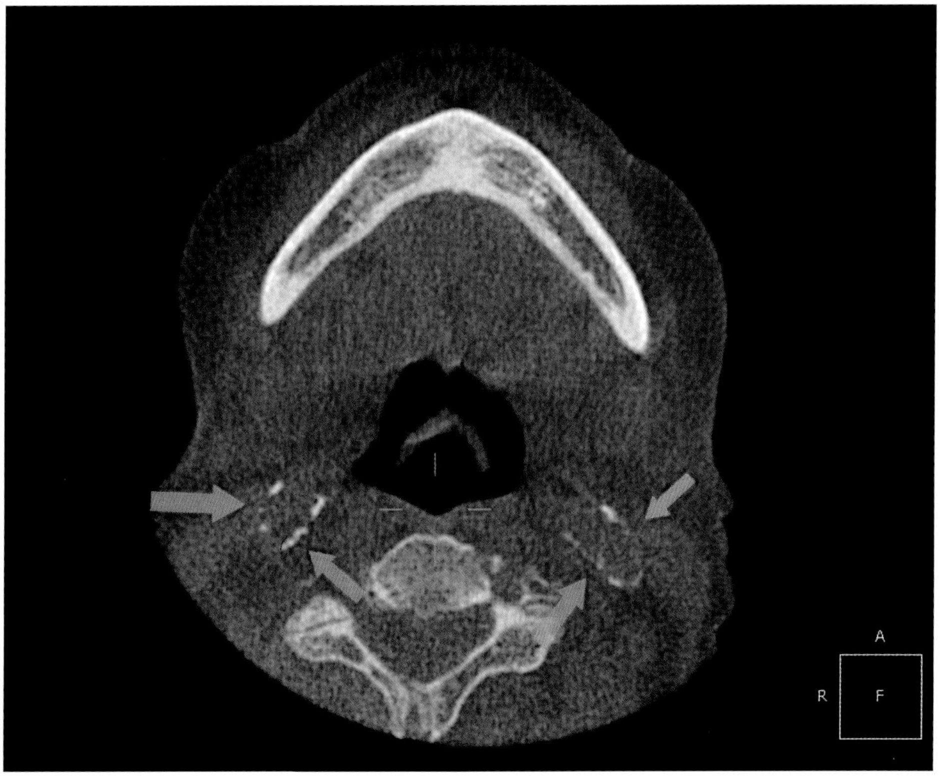

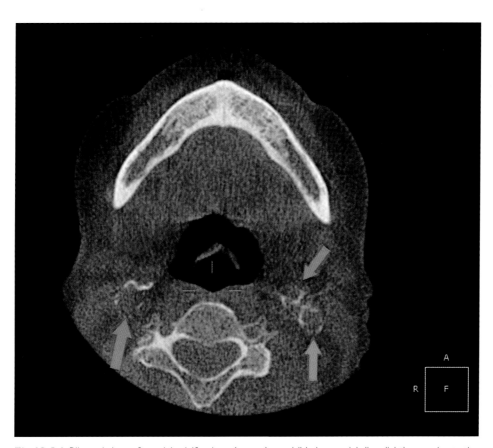

Fig 13-3c Bilateral circumferential calcifications *(arrows)* show up in this axial slice.

Fig 13-3d Bilateral circumferential calcifications *(arrows)* are visible in an axial slice slightly superior to the level in Fig 13-3c.

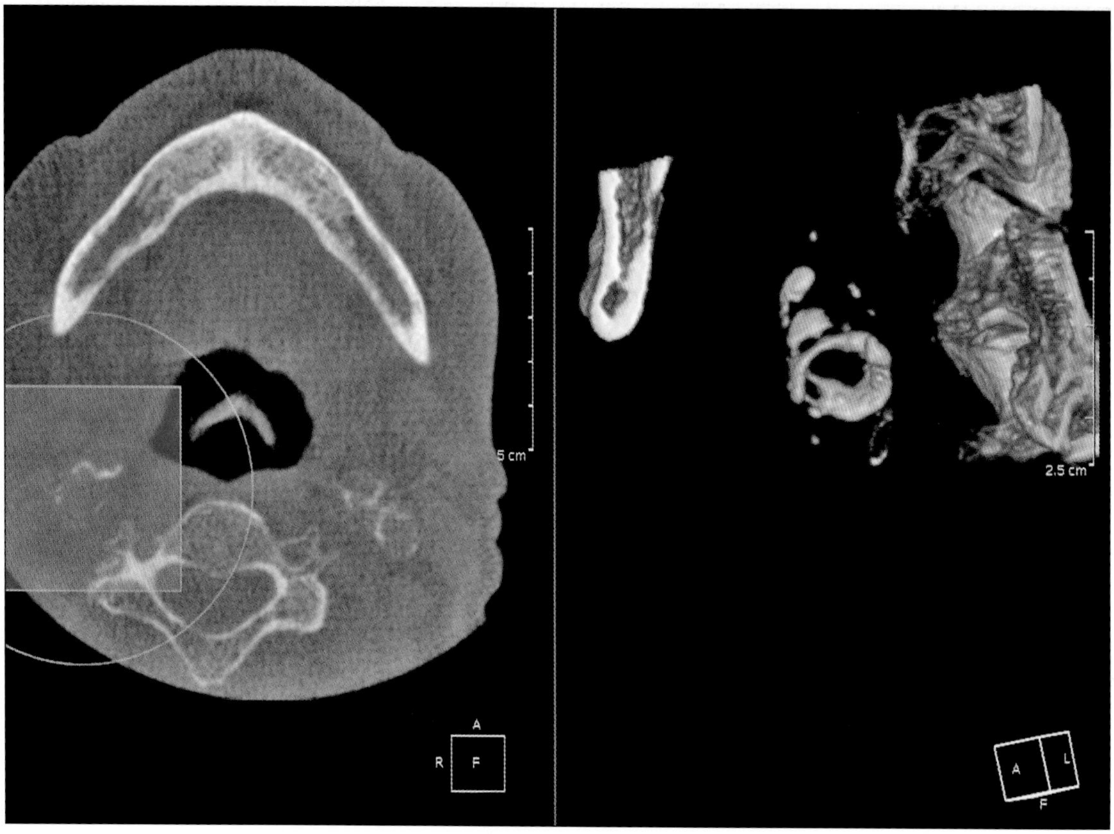

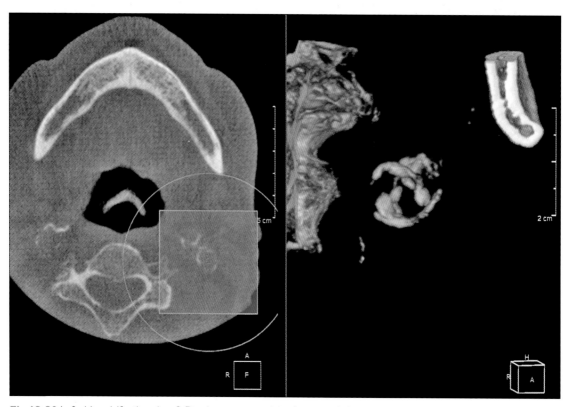

Fig 13-3e Right-side calcifications in this 3-D color reconstruction extend along a significant portion of the artery.

Fig 13-3f Left-side calcifications in a 3-D color reconstruction also extend along a significant portion of the artery.

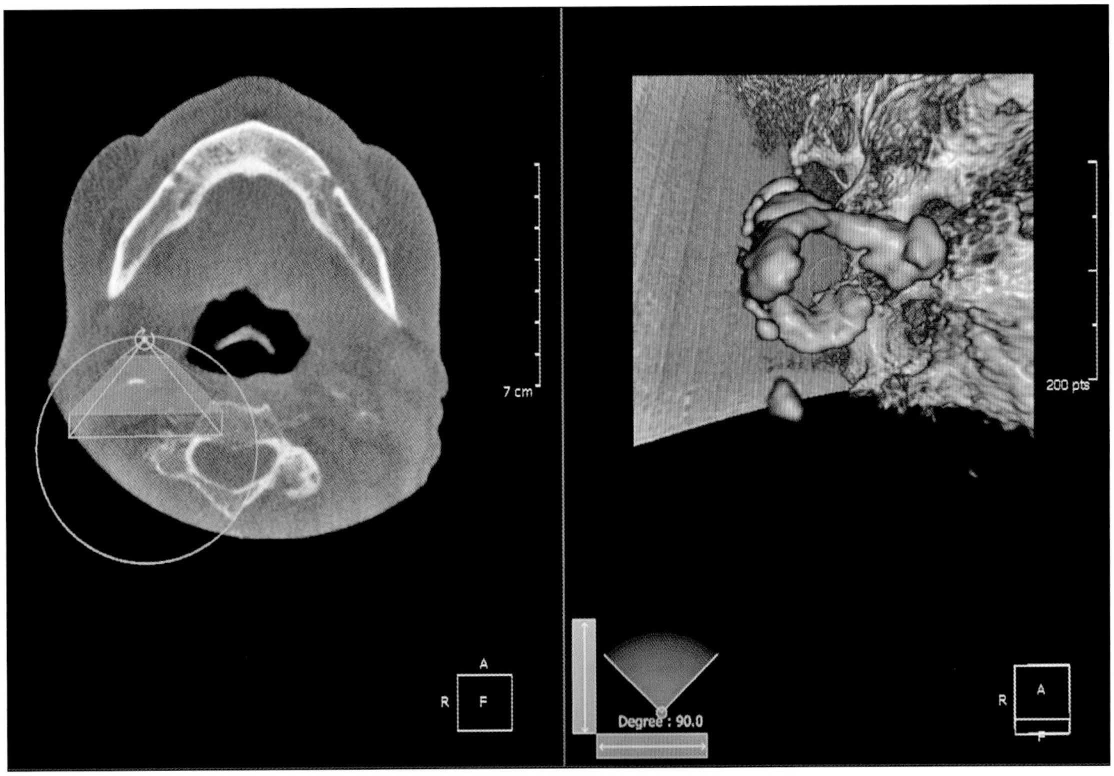

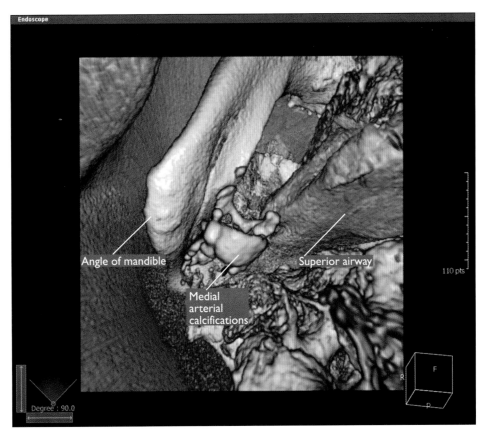

Fig 13-3g Use of the Endoscope tool in the software enhances the arterial detail.

Fig 13-3h An enlarged view provided by the Endoscope tool depicts the exact relationship of the arterial problem to the mandible and airway.

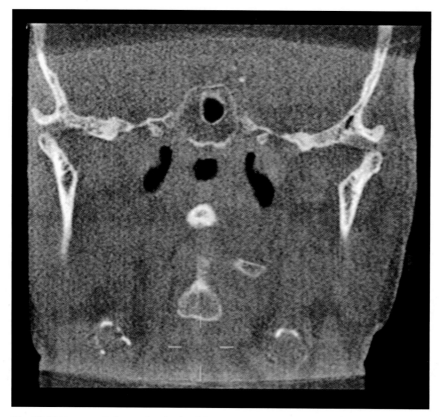

Fig 13-3i A coronal slice at the depth of the anterior edge of mandibular condyles.

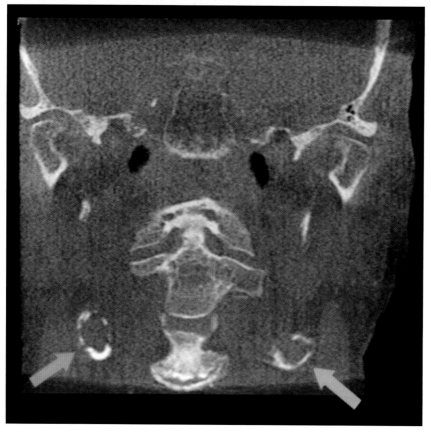

Fig 13-3j A coronal section slightly more posterior to that in Fig 13-3i shows excellent definition of the calcified arterial rings (arrows).

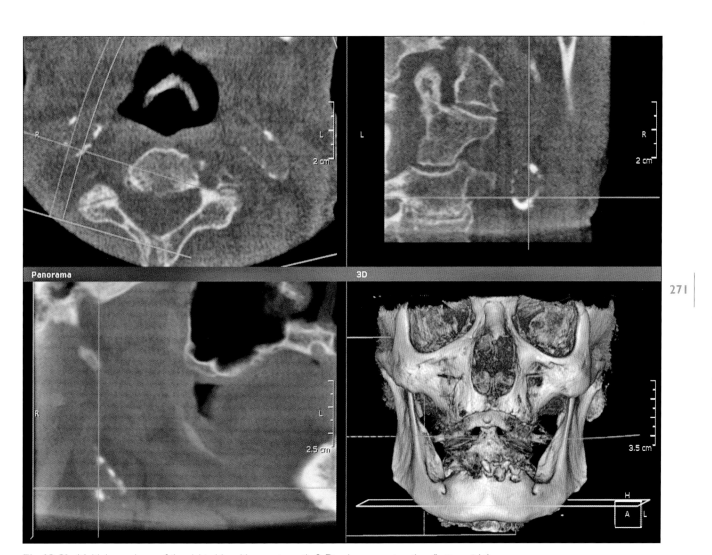

Fig 13-3k Multiplanar views of the right side with an automatic 3-D color reconstruction *(bottom right)*.

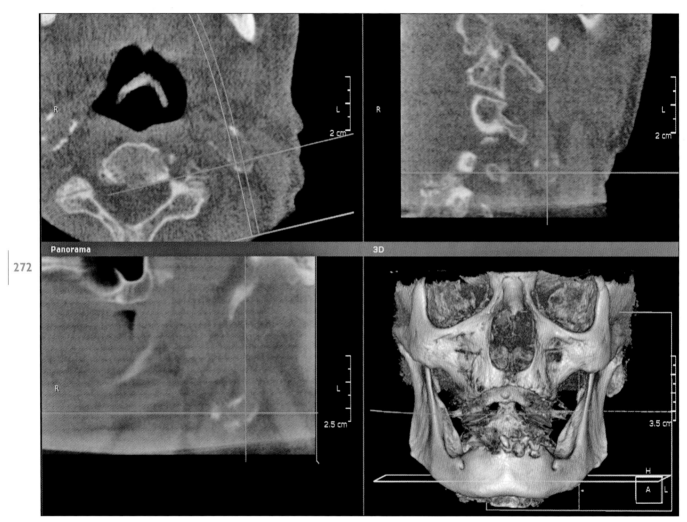

Fig 13-31 Multiplanar views of the left side with an automatic 3-D color reconstruction *(bottom right)*.

FIG

13-4

BISPHOSPHONATE-INDUCED
OSTEONECROSIS OF THE JAW

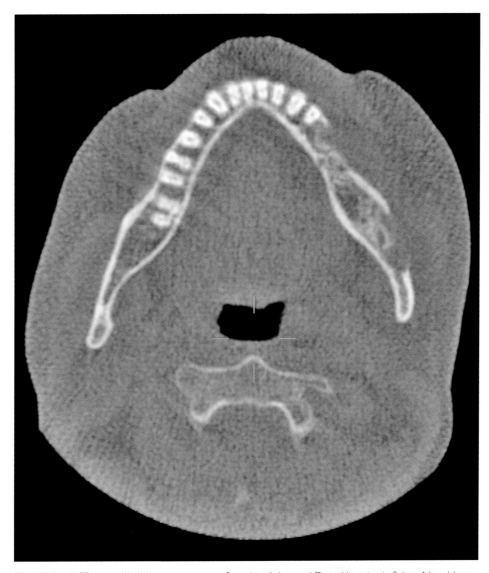

Fig 13-4a A 55-year-old white woman was referred to Advanced Dental Imaging in Salem, New Hampshire, for a cone beam scan to evaluate a previous extraction site on the left side of the posterior mandible. The imaging illustrates the diagnosis of osteonecrosis of the jaw secondary to bisphosphonate medication. A thin axial slice shows an ill-defined radiolucency in the left side of the posterior mandible. There are multiple perforative defects.

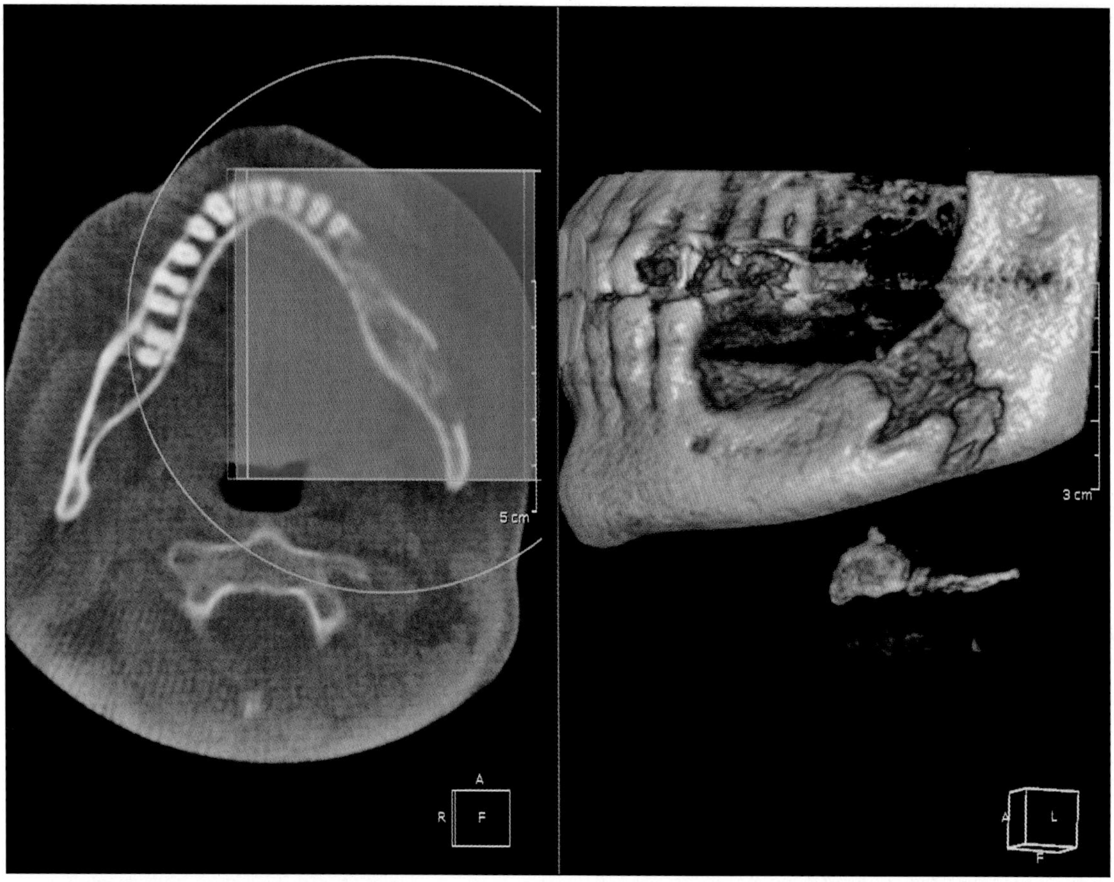

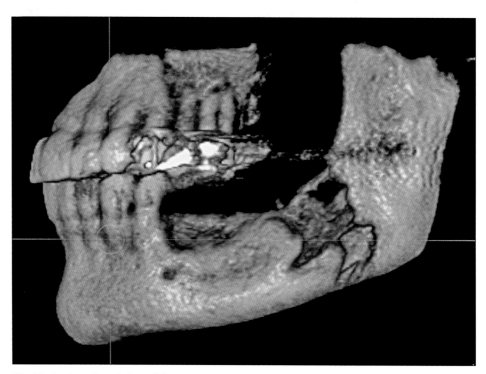

Fig 13-4b The Cube tool is used to create a 3-D color reconstruction.

Fig 13-4c An enlarged view of the reconstruction in Fig 13-4b.

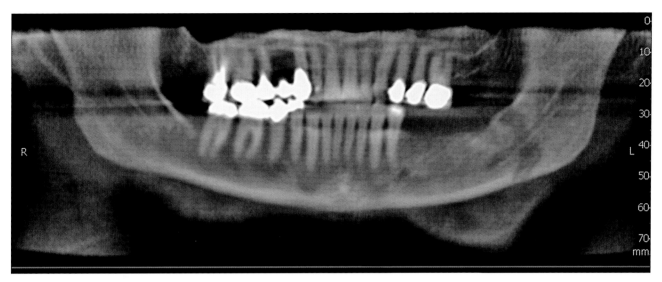

Fig 13-4d A panoramic reconstruction at a thickness of about 25 mm.

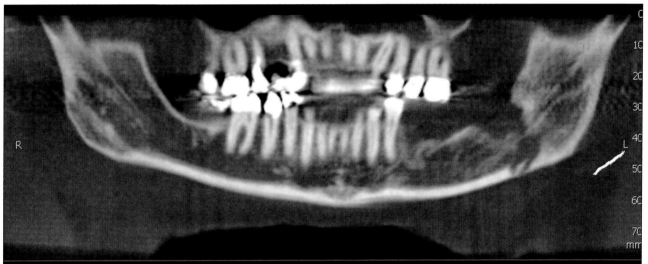

275

Fig 13-4e A pseudopanoramic reconstruction at a thickness of about 9.1 mm.

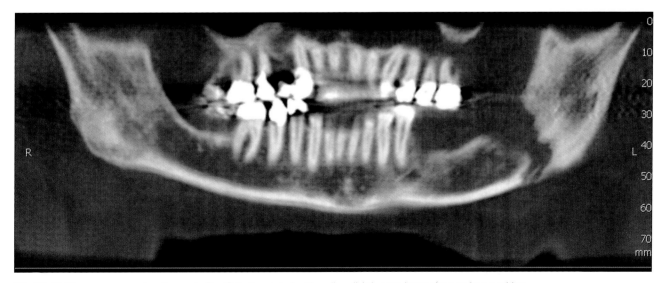

Fig 13-4f The same reconstruction as in Fig 13-4e is created with a slice slightly anterior to the previous position.

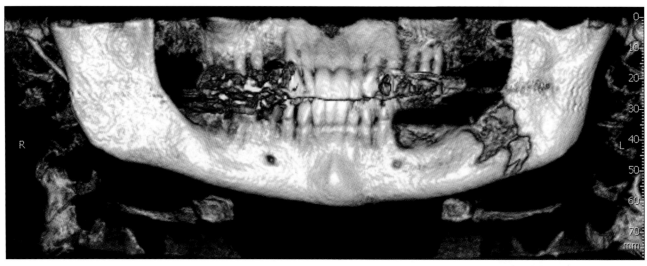

Fig 13-4g A 3-D color panoramic image shows scatter artifacts from the existing metallic restorations.

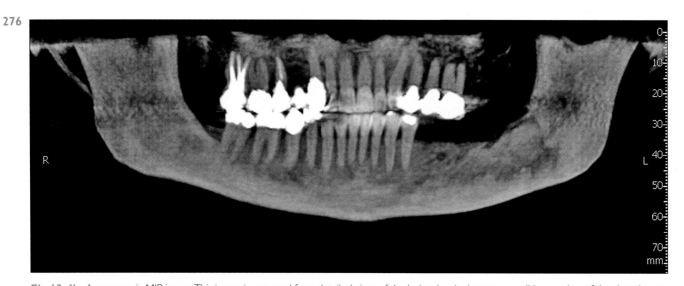

Fig 13-4h A panoramic MIP image. This image is *not* good for a detailed view of the lesion, but it gives an overall impression of the dental treatment without the scatter artifacts seen above.

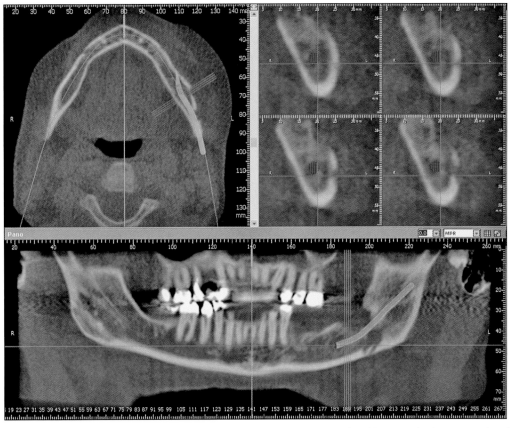

Fig 13-4i The Dental tool, used mainly for implant site assessment, is employed here to obtain cross-sectional slices *(top right)* from the anterior to the posterior of the lesion and to delineate the location of the inferior alveolar nerve *(red dot)* relative to the lesion.

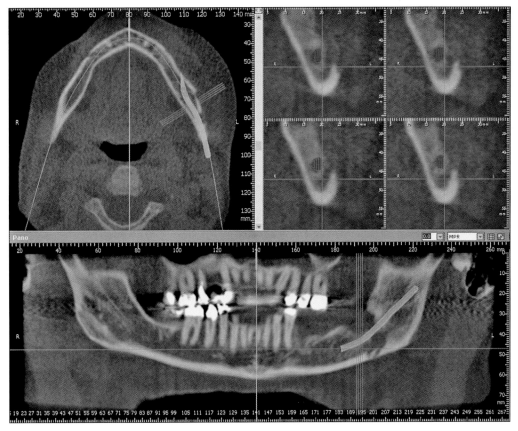

Fig 13-4j This cross-sectional slice is posterior to that in Fig 13-4i.

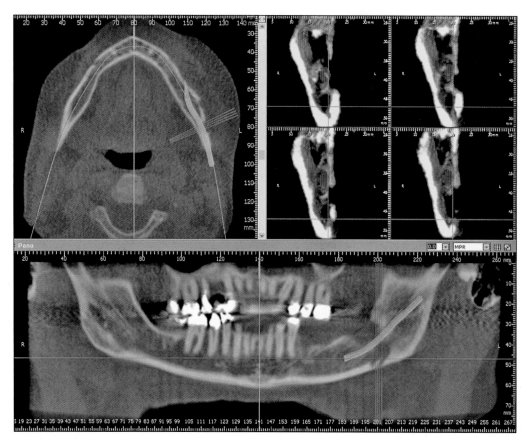

Fig 13-4k This cross-sectional slice is posterior to that in Fig 13-4j.

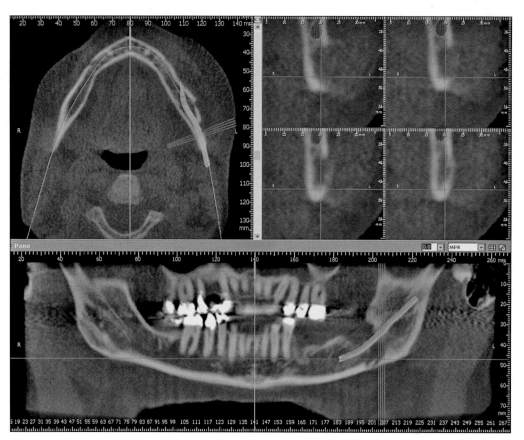

Fig 13-4l This cross-sectional slice is posterior to that in Fig 13-4k.

FIG

13-5

SQUAMOUS CELL CARCINOMA

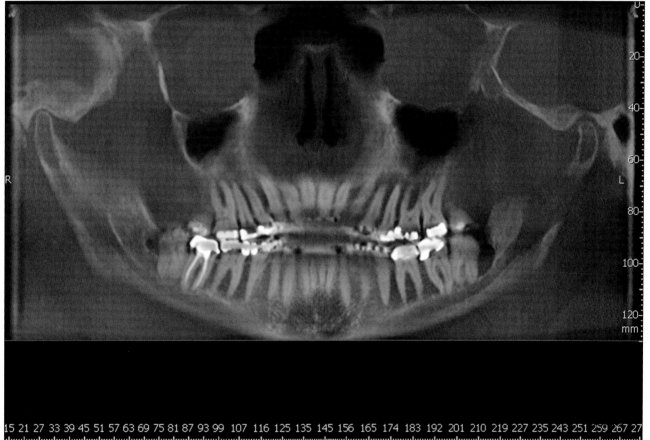

15 21 27 33 39 45 51 57 63 69 75 81 87 93 99 107 116 125 135 145 156 165 174 183 192 201 210 219 227 235 243 251 259 267 27

Fig 13-5a A 51-year-old white man was seen at an imaging center in South Dakota for evaluation of radiolucencies associated with partially impacted mandibular third molars. The mandibular left third molar was symptomatic. Whole-body positron emission tomography and computerized tomography scans identified bilateral focal hypermetabolic areas in the third molar regions. The radiologist report also noted an asymmetric increase in 2-fluoro-2-deoxy-D-glucose (FDG) uptake in the left posterior mandible that was deemed "suspicious" for focal squamous cell carcinoma. The cone beam images confirm the presence of a malignancy. A panoramic image reconstructed at a thickness of about 30 mm shows bilateral pericoronal radiolucencies. Both lesions exhibit regular cortical outlines, and neither lesion looks particularly ominous.

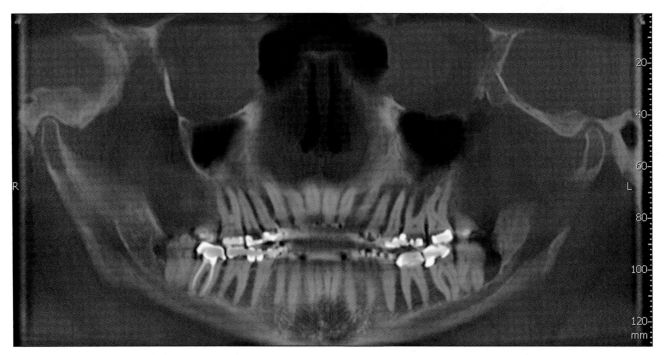

Fig 13-5b Scrolling through this panoramic image reveals that the lesion on the patient's left side appears much larger and seems to encroach on the inferior alveolar nerve canal.

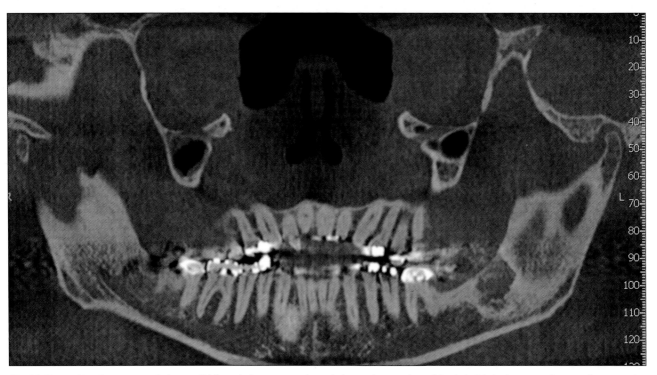

Fig 13-5c A thin slice panoramic image (0.15 mm) shows some irregularity at the margins of the left-side lesion, as well as small permeative defects. These are more ominous radiographic features.

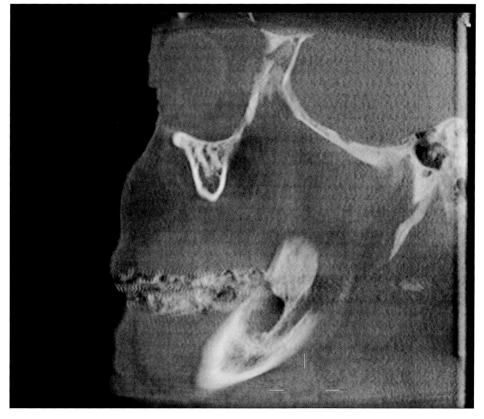

Fig 13-5d A sagittal view shows the proximity of the left-side lesion to the nerve canal.

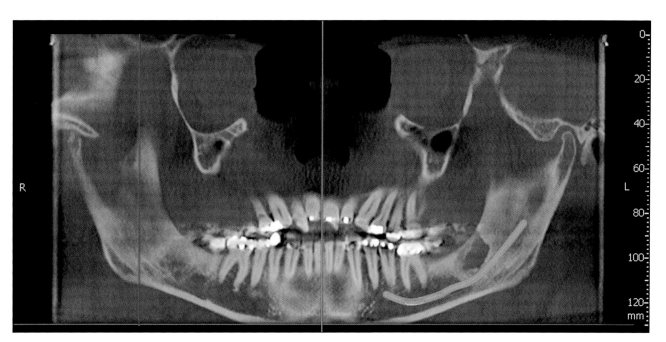

Fig 13-5e By using the Dental tool, which is most often reserved for implant assessment, it is possible to colorize the inferior alveolar nerve canal (green), show the proximity of the lesion to the canal, and assist the surgeon's approach.

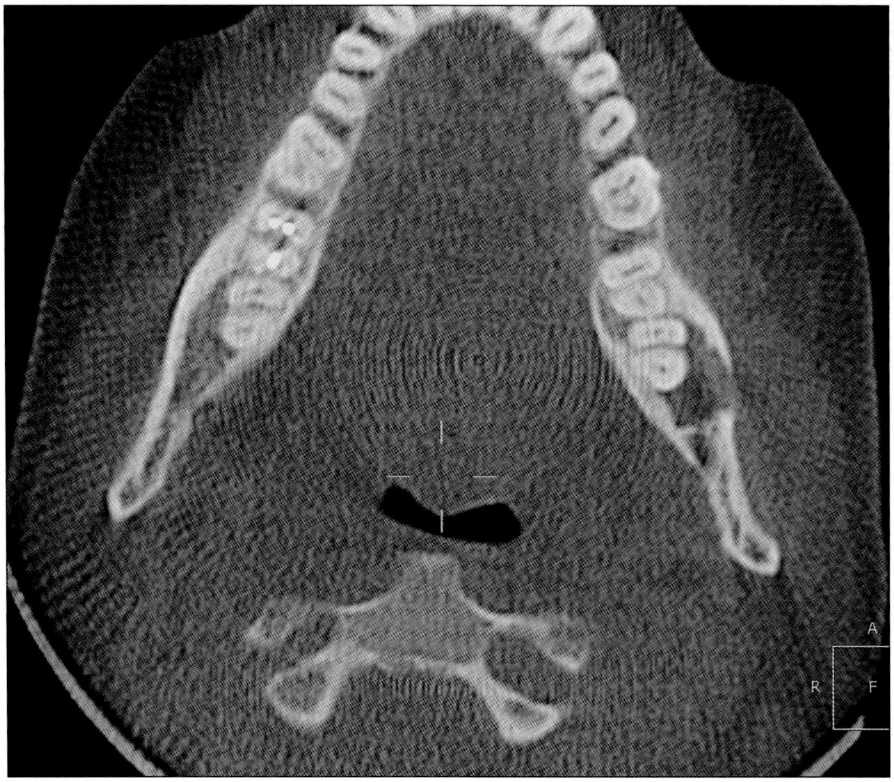

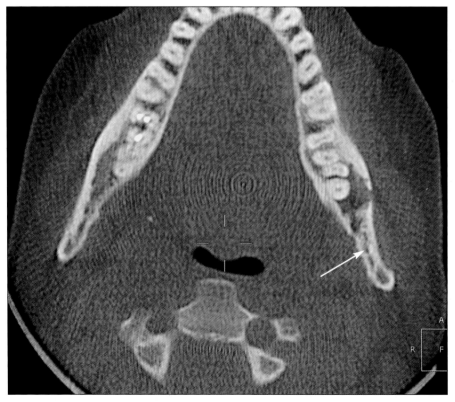

Fig 13-5f A thin axial slice (0.15 mm) shows the lesion perforating the buccal cortical bone.

Fig 13-5g A thin axial slice (0.15 mm) shows the lesion perforating the buccal cortical bone, but more importantly, it shows the permeative appearance of this lesion. The inferior alveolar nerve canal is shown by the *white arrow*.

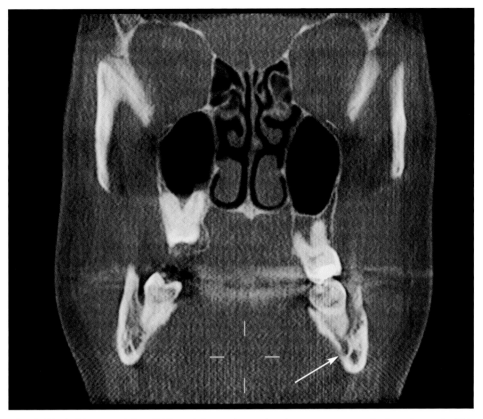

Fig 13-5h A thin coronal slice (0.15 mm) shows the permeative appearance on the buccal aspect of this lesion. The inferior alveolar nerve canal is shown by the *white arrow*.

283

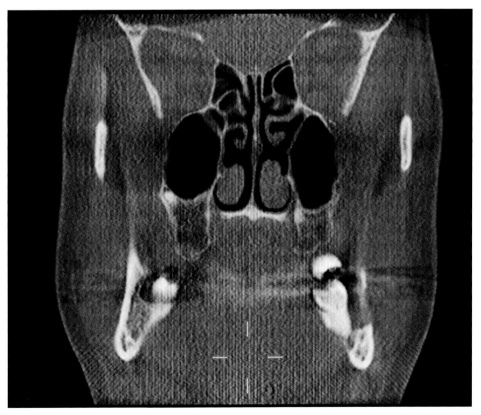

Fig 13-5i A more posterior coronal slice reveals destroyed cortical bone. Note the intact marginal area on the mandibular right third molar.

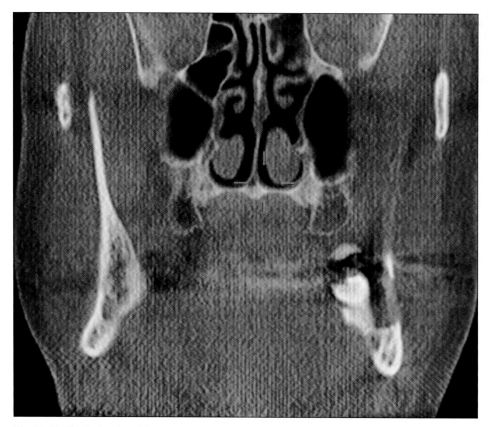

Fig 13-5j This is the site of the greatest cortical destruction.

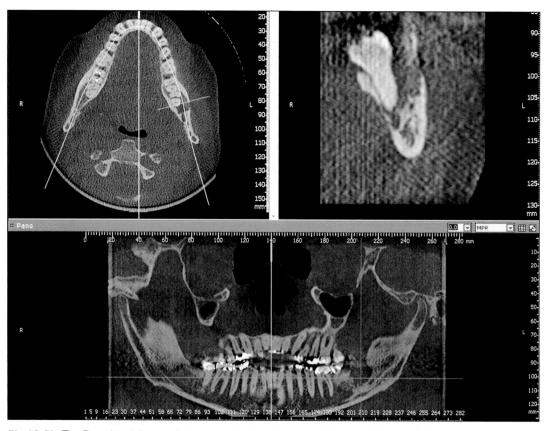

Fig 13-5k The Dental tool shows axial, cross-sectional, and panoramic images relating the lesion appearance.

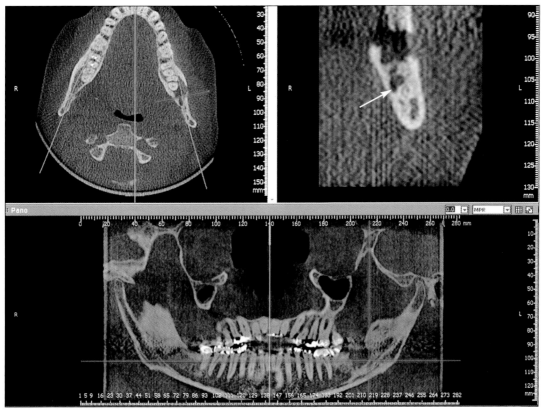

Fig 13-5l The Dental tool shows axial, cross-sectional, and panoramic images at the most posterior aspect of the lesion. The nerve canal (*arrow*) appears to be separate from the lesion at this point.

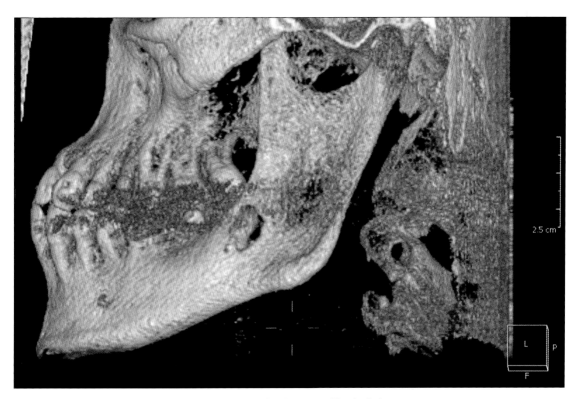

Fig 13-5m A 3-D color reconstruction shows the perforation caused by the lesion.

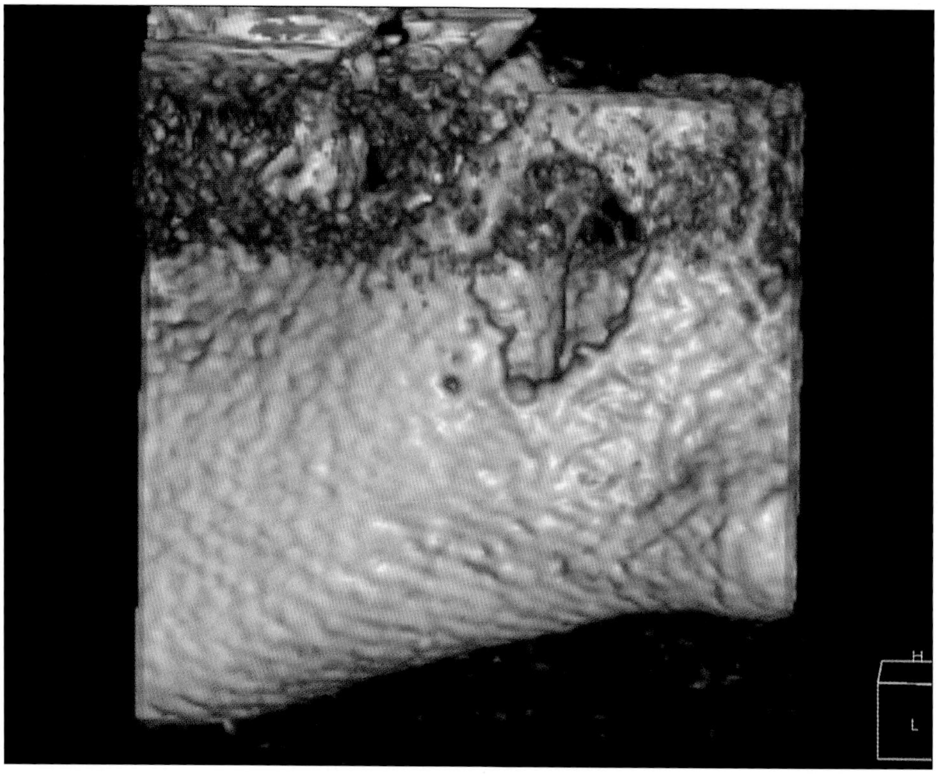

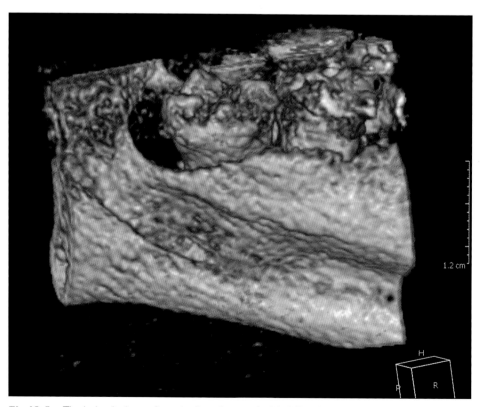

Fig 13-5n A close-up 3-D color reconstruction provides a detailed look at the perforation.

Fig 13-5o The lesion is shown from the lingual aspect in this 3-D color reconstruction.

REFERENCES

1. Friedlander AH, Baker JD. Panoramic radiography: An aid in detecting patients at risk of cerebrovascular accident. J Am Dent Assoc 1994;125:1598–1603.

2. Friedlander AH. Identification of stroke-prone patients by panoramic and cervical spine radiography. Dentomaxillofac Radiol 1995;24:160–164.

3. Carter LC, Tsimidis K, Fabiano J. Carotid calcifications on panoramic radiography identify an asymptomatic male patient at risk for stroke. A case report. Oral Surg Oral Med Oral Pathol Oral Radiol Endod 1998;85:119–122.

4. Amos AF, McCarty DJ, Zimmet P. The rising global burden of diabetes and its complications: Estimates and projections to the year 2010. Diabet Med 1997;14(suppl 5):S1–S85.

5. National Diabetes Education Program. Working together to manage diabetes: A guide for pharmacy, podiatry, optometry, and dental professionals, 2007. Available at: http://www.ndep.nih.gov/diabetes/WTMD/index.htm. Accessed 8 August 2008.

6. Miles DA, Craig RM, Langlais RP, Wadsworth WC. Facial artery calcification: A case report of its clinical significance. J Can Dent Assoc 1983;49:200–202.

7. Miles DA, Craig RM. The calcified facial artery. A report of the panoramic radiographic incidence and appearance. Oral Surg Oral Med Oral Pathol 1983; 55:214–219.

8. Augustine J, Vidt DG. Cleveland Clinic Disease Management Project: Diabetic nephropathy. Available at: http://www.clevelandclinicmeded.com/medicalpubs/diseasemanagement/nephrology/diabeticnephropathy/diabeticnephropathy.htm#prevalence. Accessed 8 August 2008.

9. Hayden MR, Tyagi SC, Kolb L, Sowers JR, Khanna R. Vascular ossification–calcification in metabolic syndrome, type 2 diabetes mellitus, chronic kidney disease, and calciphylaxis–calcific uremic arteriolopathy: The emerging role of sodium thiosulfate. Cardiovasc Diabetol 2005;4(1):4.

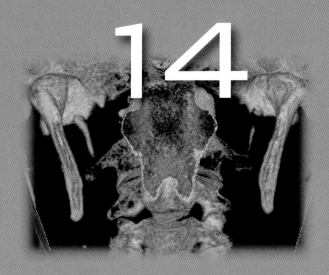

14

VERTEBRAL BODY EVALUATION

A joint is a joint is a joint . . . or so I used to teach my graduate students. Although the temporomandibular joint (TMJ) is specialized in its motion capability and the mandible is the only bone in the body with an articulation on each side, the TMJs are considered "loaded" just like the knees and hips and can demonstrate comparable osteoarthritic changes. On plain radiographs or even digital images, many condyles that are "ugly," misshapen, modified by osteophytic activity, or even grossly altered in their morphology still might be totally asymptomatic. On the other hand, using these same image receptors (eg, panoramic, tomographic), TMJs may appear normal and yet be quite painful. The pain, especially in conditions like osteoarthritis (OA), might precede the actual radiographic change by many months. Now, with cone beam volumetric imaging (CBVI), we may have an opportunity to detect the osteoarthritic changes earlier. There can be a correlation to other loaded joints like the knee and/or intervertebral joints as well. When I see vertebral bodies with subchondral cyst formation and subchondral sclerosis in cone beam images, I also often see concomitant changes on the condylar head. In Table 1-1, 32 of the 381 total patients were found to have osteoarthritic changes in the vertebrae. That represents approximately 8.4% of that initial patient population.

FIG
14-1

OSTEOARTHRITIC FINDINGS: CASE 1

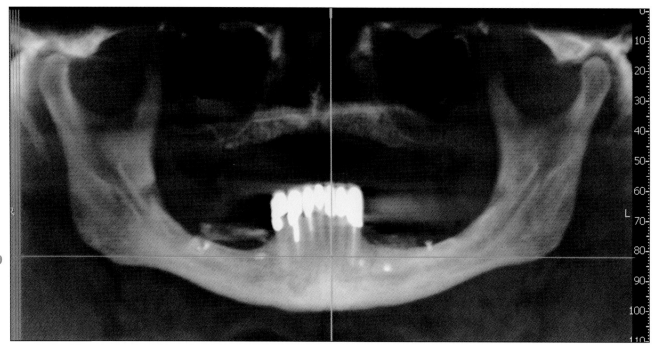

290

Fig 14-1a This patient showed significant changes in the cervical vertebrae without major alteration of the TMJ condyles. Unlike rheumatoid arthritis, which is polyarticular and symmetric and can affect the condyles, OA usually affects one or two major loaded joints in the body asymmetrically. A panoramic reconstruction shows ostensibly normal condyles.

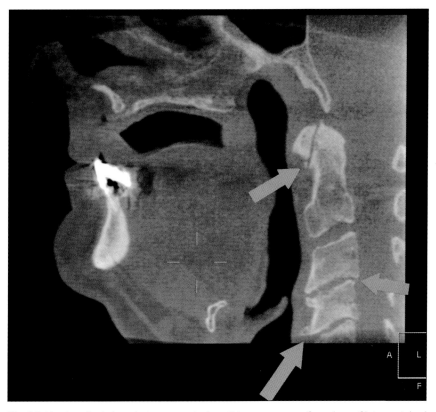

Fig 14-1b A sagittal view shows osteophytic activity on many surfaces, loss of intervertebral joint space, and subluxation of the vertebrae C3 to C5 *(arrows)*.

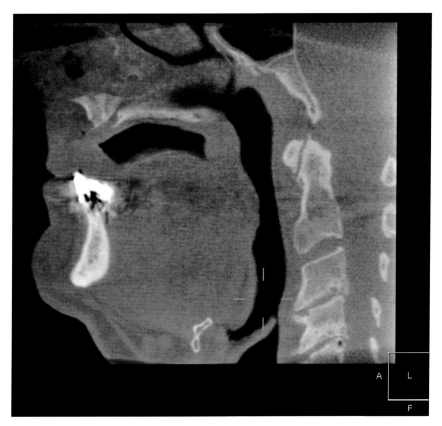

Fig 14-1c This sagittal view reveals significant subchondral sclerosis and subchondral cyst formation on C3 to C5.

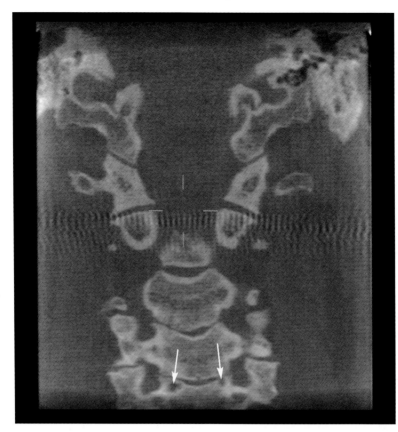

Fig 14-1d A coronal view shows the subchondral cysts on C5 *(arrows)*.

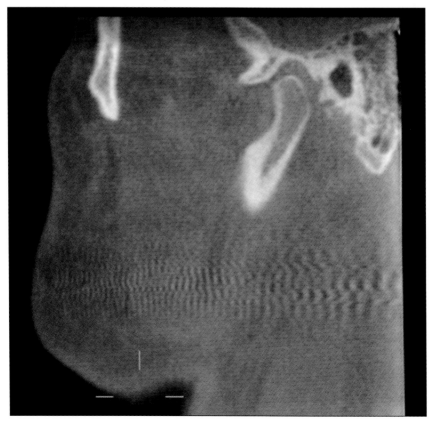

Fig 14-1e The right condylar head appears normal in this thin sagittal slice (0.15 mm).

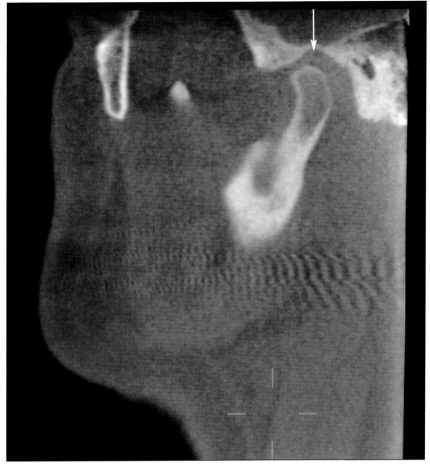

Fig 14-1f The left condylar head may have a slight cortical thickening (arrow), which is indicative of early subchondral sclerosis.

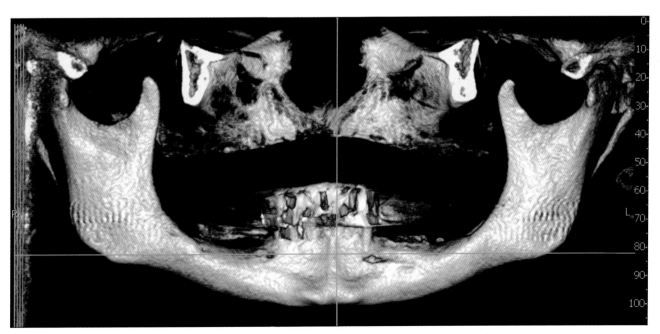

Fig 14-1g A 3-D color panoramic reconstruction demonstrates that the condyles, although altered slightly in shape, appear normal.

FIG

14-2

OSTEOARTHRITIC FINDINGS: CASE 2

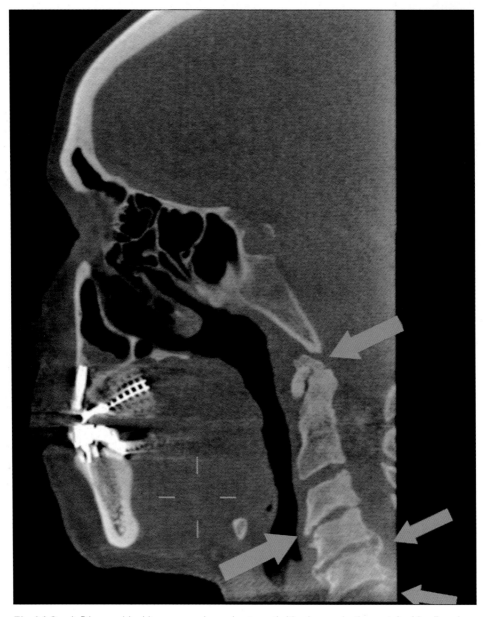

Fig 14-2a A 56-year-old white woman showed osteoarthritic changes in the vertebral bodies, along with slight concomitant condylar head involvement. There are significant osteophytic changes on C3, C4, and C5, with collapse of the intervertebral joint spaces and subluxation *(bottom three arrows)*. C2 also shows subchondral sclerosis and possible fusion with the anterior arch of C1 *(top arrow)*.

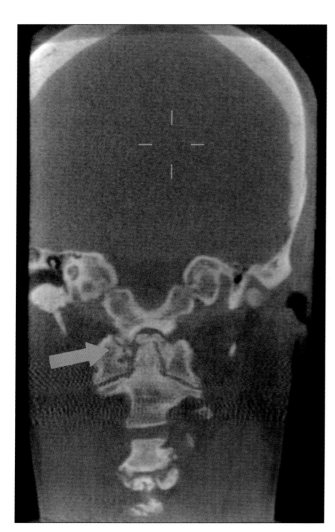

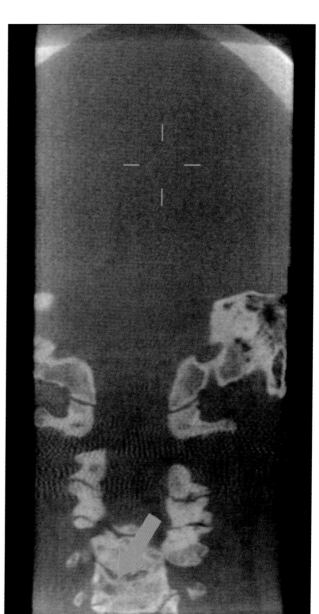

Fig 14-2b Subchondral cyst formation on C1.

Fig 14-2c Additional subchondral cyst formation *(arrow)*.

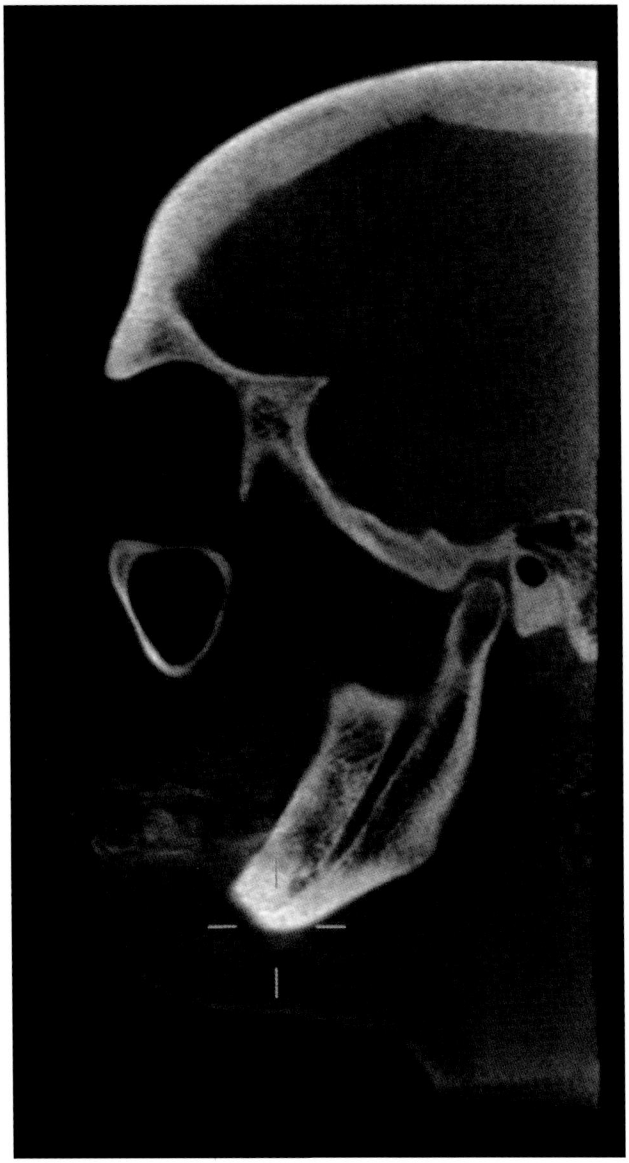

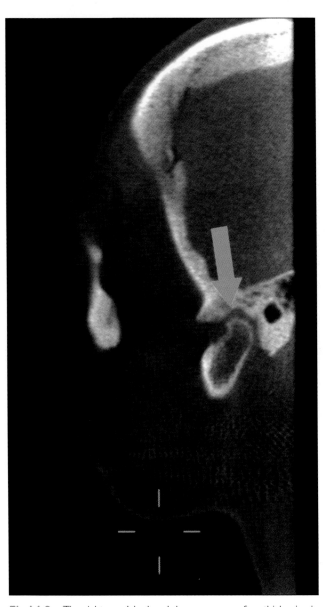

Fig 14-2d The left condylar head appears normal.

Fig 14-2e The right condylar head shows some surface thickening in the form of subchondral sclerosis *(arrow)*. This is an early change but indicative of synovial fluid loss and subsequent bone formation to protect the condylar surface.

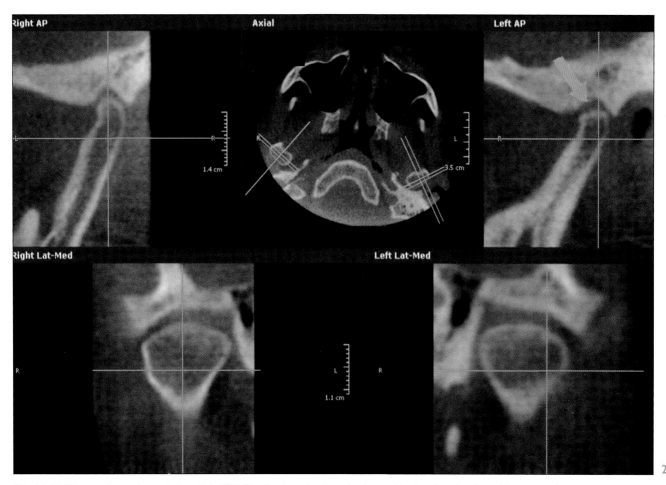

Fig 14-2f Direct volumetric rendering of the TMJ. The Dual mode allows both condylar heads to be viewed for comparison.

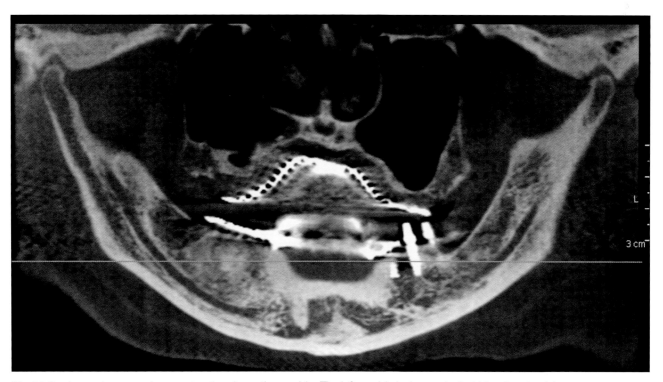

Fig 14-2g A pseudopanoramic reconstruction shows the condyles. The left condyle looks marginally thicker than the right.

FIG

14-3

OSTEOARTHRITIC FINDINGS: CASE 3

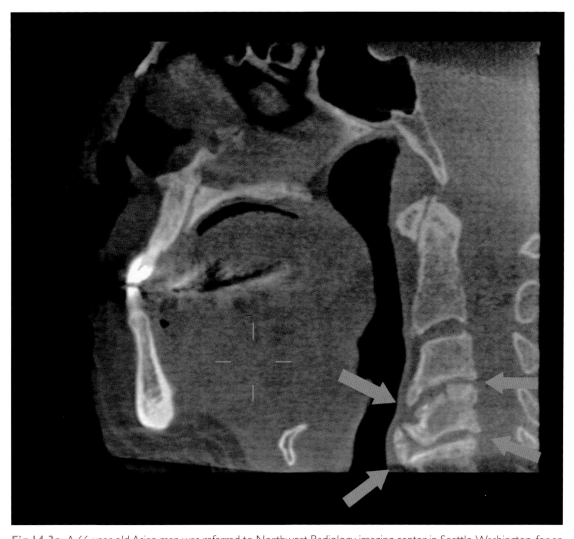

Fig 14-3a A 66-year-old Asian man was referred to Northwest Radiology imaging center in Seattle, Washington, for an implant site assessment. Osteoarthritic findings are apparent, with severe osteophyte formation, subluxation, and loss of intervertebral joint space seen on C3, C4, and C5 *(arrows)*. There is also a large erosion on the anterior aspect of C4 *(upper left arrow)*.

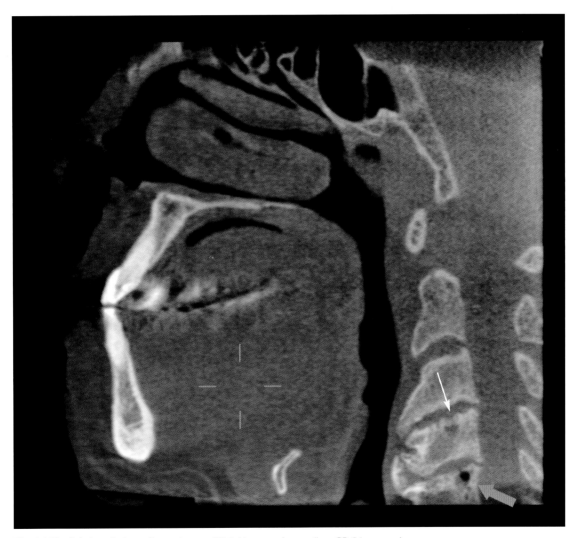

Fig 14-3b Subchondral cyst formation on C4 *(white arrow)* as well as C5 *(blue arrow).*

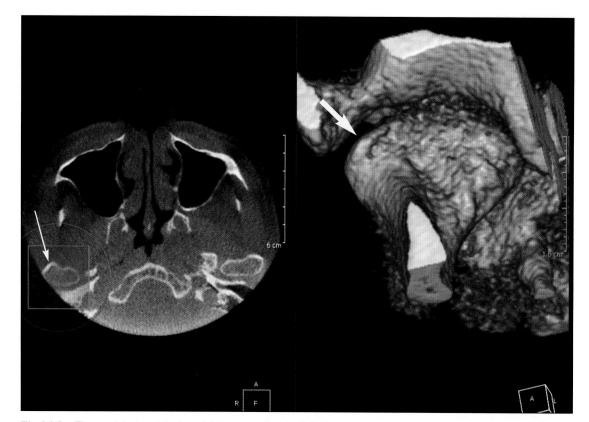

Fig 14-3c The condylar heads in the axial view, as well as the 3-D Cube tool color reconstruction of the right condyle, appear relatively normal. *(left)* Some slight cortical thickening may be present on the lateral pole *(small arrow)* in the axial view. *(right)* The 3-D reconstruction shows it to be condylar lipping *(large arrow)*.

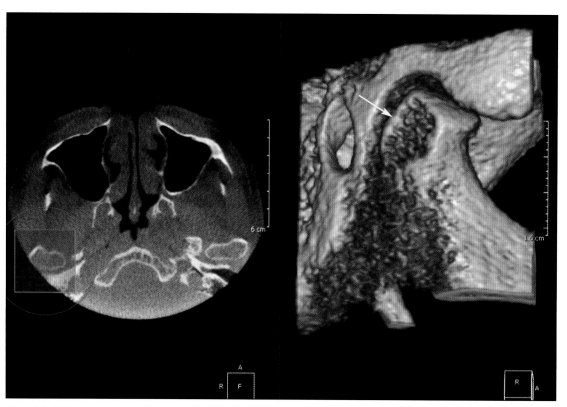

Fig 14-3d The right condyle in 3-D color is rotated to show the lateral aspect. The deep depression *(arrow)* is an imaging artifact; the patient was not correctly positioned to capture the entire condylar area.

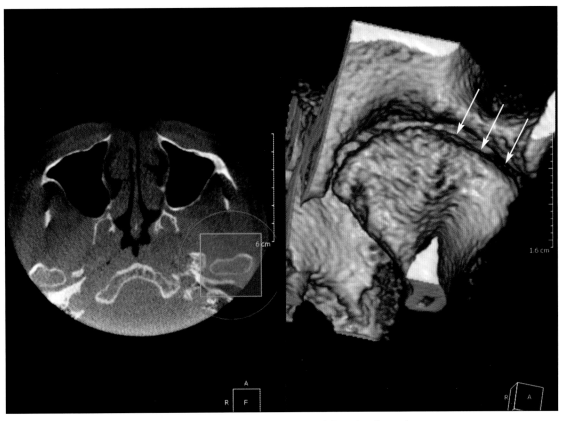

Fig 14-3e The left condyle is essentially normal except for some mild flattening *(arrows)*.

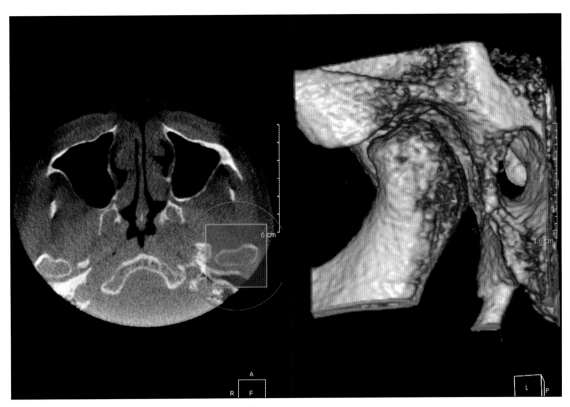

Fig 14-3f Lateral aspect of the left condyle seen in Fig 14-3e.

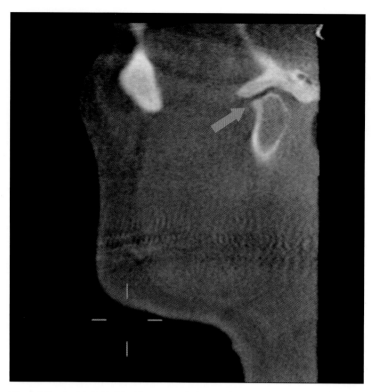

Fig 14-3g In this 2-D thin slice grayscale image, the anterior portion of the left condyle *(blue arrow)* looks like an osteophytic projection. However, the 3-D color rendering in Fig 14-3f shows that this shape is just the result of some flattening of the condyle.

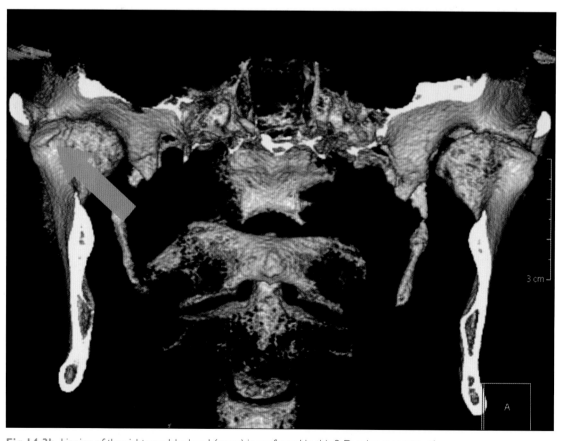

Fig 14-3h Lipping of the right condylar head *(arrow)* is confirmed in this 3-D color reconstruction.

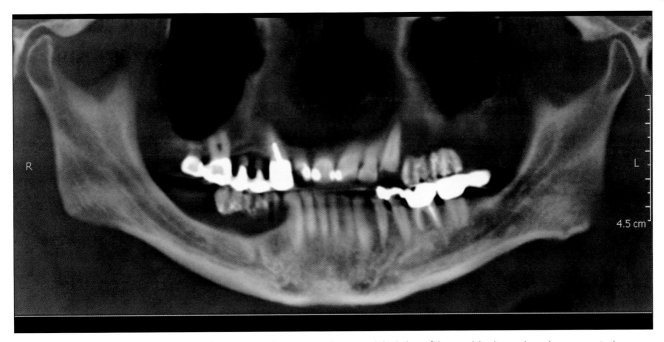

Fig 14-3i Even though this 3-D color panoramic reconstruction suggests an osteophytic projection with the traditional bird-beak appearance (*arrow*), it has been shown that this is actually flattening and lipping of the condylar surface. Regardless of appearance, the condition can still be attributed to OA.

Fig 14-3j Although this grayscale panoramic reconstruction seems to be a good depiction of the condyles, it grossly underrepresents the scope of condylar change seen in the previous images of this case.

INDEX

305